Female sterilization

A guide to provision of services

WORLD HEALTH ORGANIZATION
GENEVA
1992

WHO Library Cataloguing in Publication Data

Female sterilization : a guide to provision of services.

1.Family planning 2.Sterilization, Sexual I.Title
ISBN 92 4 154434 1 (NLM Classification: WP 660)

TYPESET IN INDIA
PRINTED IN ENGLAND

90/8711 – Macmillan/Clays/GCW – 6000

Contents

Preface

The primary purpose of these guidelines is to assist those responsible for the development and management of family planning and health programmes in initiating or expanding female sterilization services. This book is designed to serve the needs of various types of personnel, including managers, administrators, and service providers. It shows how to extend the accessibility of female sterilization through different types of services and delivery channels, and how to develop awareness of it as a contraceptive option. Basic technical information about tubal occlusion, its effects, and related medical issues is included so that service staff will have the necessary background and understanding. Although this publication is not intended to be a manual for training in the surgical techniques of female sterilization, it includes information that will be useful to those responsible for establishing and administering training programmes for female sterilization.

Every attempt has been made to make these guidelines of practical value for those who are establishing female sterilization services. Thus, chapters on organizing and managing services and on financial management and budgeting are included, along with several annexes that provide sample materials that can be adapted to local needs.

These guidelines are particularly timely because of the growing interest in and demand for female sterilization services in many parts of the world. The views summarized here represent a consensus of the members of an expert group that met in Rio de Janeiro in October 1988, and of experts from around the world who have reviewed the manuscript, including the review group that met in New Delhi in December 1991. The guidelines are meant to be flexible: the aim is to present important issues and to make suggestions that can be readily adapted to specific services within the social and cultural context of each country.

These guidelines are part of a series of technical publications on family planning that have been issued by the World Health Organization since 1976 (see inside back cover).

Comments and queries on this publication should be addressed to: Maternal and Child Health and Family Planning, Division of Family Health, World Health Organization, 1211 Geneva 27, Switzerland.

Acknowledgements

The World Health Organization acknowledges the help of the Association for Voluntary Surgical Contraception (AVSC) in the preparation of these guidelines, in particular: Mr T. W. Jezowski, Director of International Programs; Dr D. H. Huber, Medical Director; Ms P. Harper, Publications Manager; and Ms S. C. Huber, Consultant. Dr H. Hoogenboom, Executive Director and Dr A. E. Pollack, Medical Director, also provided valuable assistance.

Many valuable comments were received from the expert group that met in Rio de Janeiro. The participants were: Dr M. Belsey, WHO, Geneva; Professor W. O. Chukudebelu, Nigeria; Dr A. M. Dourlen, Rollier, France; Dr M. Fathalla, WHO, Geneva; Dr A. Faundes, Brazil; Dr J. Githiari, Kenya; Professor V. Hingorani, India; Dr Hua Jhia Zhen, China; Dr C. Huezo, England; Dr R. Jacobstein, United States of America; Dr Z. Khairullah, United States of America; Dr D. Mastrorocco, Brazil; Dr L. Mehra, WHO, Geneva; Dr Chan Moo Park, Republic of Korea; Dr I. O. Otolorin, Nigeria; Dr R. Santiso, Guatemala; Dr P. Senanayake, England; Dr R. Soonawala, India; Professor Yan Renying, China; Dr A. Yuzpe, Canada.

Thanks are also due to the review group that met in New Delhi: Dr R. Baveja, India; Dr V. Kumar, WHO Regional Office for South-East Asia, New Delhi, India; Dr L. Mehra, WHO, Geneva; Dr S. Mehta, WHO, Geneva; Dr S. N. Mukerjee, India. The manuscript was also reviewed by the following people, whose contribution is gratefully acknowledged: Ms B. S. Atkins, World Federation of Health Agencies for the Advancement of Voluntary Surgical Contraception; Dr M. R. Couper, WHO, Geneva; Dr M. B. Dobson, Oxford, England; Dr D. V. I. Fairweather, International Federation of Gynecology and Obstetrics; Dr E. Kessel, International Federation of Gynecology and Obstetrics; Dr A. Rahman Khan, United Nations Population Fund; Dr M. H. Khayat, WHO Regional Office for the Eastern Mediterranean, Alexandria, Egypt; Dr D. Pierotti,

WHO Regional Office for Europe, Copenhagen, Denmark; Mr J. M. Pile, World Federation of Health Agencies for the Advancement of Voluntary Surgical Contraception; Professor S. S. Ratnam, Singapore; Professor M. Rauff, Singapore; Ms S. Schneider, Program for Appropriate Technology in Health; Dr J. Sciarra, United States of America; Dr P. Senanayake, International Planned Parenthood Federation; Dr P. Severyns, United Nations Population Fund; Dr M. Trías, Colombia; Dr L. Tyrer, United States of America; and Dr A. E. Wasunna, WHO, Geneva.

The financial and technical support of the United Nations Population Fund (UNFPA) is also gratefully acknowledged.

1. General considerations

Introduction

Female sterilization is the most widely used contraceptive method in the world today. Over 100 million women of child-bearing age have been sterilized, and it is estimated that more than 100 million women in the developing world alone will seek sterilization in the next 20 years.

Female sterilization, which is also called tubal ligation or tubal occlusion, is a relatively straightforward surgical procedure in which the fallopian tubes are permanently occluded in order to prevent fertilization (see Fig. 1).

When correctly performed, female sterilization is highly effective and safe. In many cases the procedure may be carried out on an outpatient basis under local anaesthesia. However, as with any surgical procedure, certain risks are involved. The operation must, therefore, be performed by trained personnel in appropriate service-delivery settings and under conditions where medical quality can be assured. Nevertheless, an elaborate medical setting and expensive equipment are not essential.

Female sterilization may be an attractive contraceptive choice for couples who want no more children. However, because it is intended to be permanent, involves the risks associated with surgery, and has a small possibility of failure, it should be ensured that clients choosing female sterilization are making a fully informed voluntary decision. Other methods of contraception must also be available, without pressure or inducements, and information and counselling must be offered.

These guidelines are intended to help service providers and managers set up and maintain high-quality female sterilization services. Such services should be voluntary, medically safe and effective, appropriate to the health care setting, respectful of clients, and well managed and efficient. Attention to quality is the key to client satisfaction and success.

Fig. 1. Female sterilization

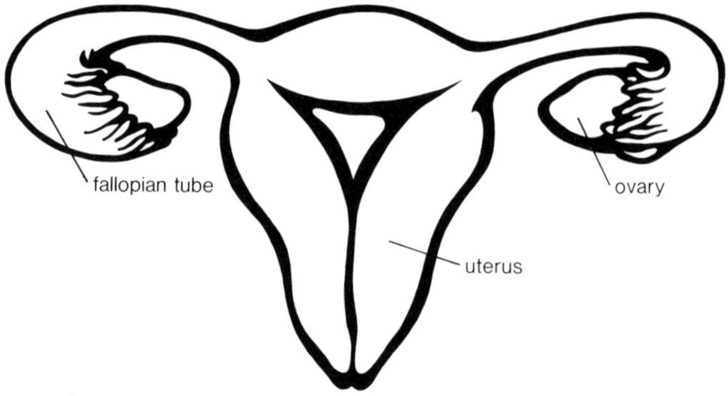

Before sterilization

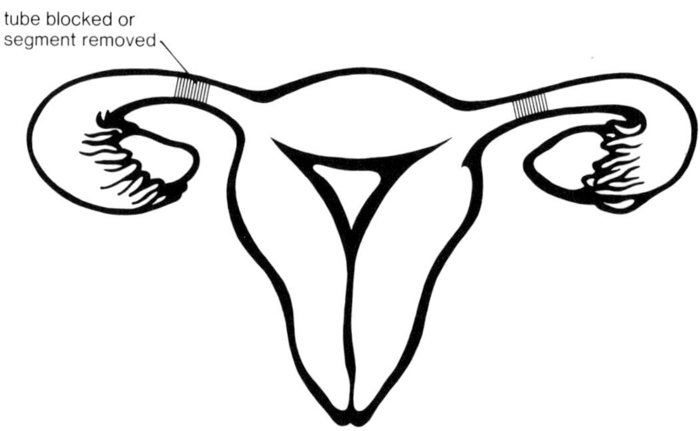

After sterilization

The role of female sterilization in regulating fertility

Female sterilization is one of several contraceptive options that can be provided through family planning, primary health, and maternal and child health care services. It should be available as one option to women or couples who have decided that they have had the number of children they want. In many countries this decision is often made by women less than 30 years of age (Ross et al., 1985). For these women the prospect of several more years of reproductive capability may lead them to choose a fertility control method that is either permanent or long-acting.

For couples who have decided to end childbearing, sterilization for either the male or the female partner should be made available, in addition to long-lasting temporary methods (intrauterine devices, injectables, and implants) and other contraceptive choices. The availability of a wide range of contraceptive methods means that couples are more likely to find a method that suits them and hence, to plan their families. Couples should, therefore, have access to accurate information about all the methods available, including their characteristics, effects, benefits, and risks.

Health considerations

As a contraceptive method, female sterilization has both health benefits and risks. The health considerations are discussed briefly below.

Health benefits of family planning

The practice of family planning through the use of any contraceptive method provides health benefits, especially when one considers the morbidity and mortality associated with frequent pregnancy. Complications of pregnancy, childbirth, and abortion are a major cause of death among women of childbearing age throughout the world. Maternal mortality rates range from 300 to 800 per 100 000 births in developing countries (Starrs, 1987). In developed countries the average rate is 30 per 100 000 births (Ross et al., 1988). Women of high parity (three or more children) and those 30 years of age or older experience higher rates of maternal morbidity and mortality than do lower-parity and younger women (Maine, 1981). The risks associated with pregnancy are decreased for all women who practise family planning because of the pregnancies that are averted as a result. Experience suggests that, on a global basis, sterilization prevents an average of 1.5–2.5 births per woman (Ross et al., 1985), and thus the reduction in risk may be substantial.

Family size and maternal age also affect infant and childhood morbidity and mortality. Fetal and infant death rates increase with birth order, as does the incidence of low birth weight and its attendant problems. Children born to older mothers have a higher risk of birth defects and fetal and neonatal death rates are higher for mothers over 30 years of age than for women in their 20s (Maine, 1981; Puffer & Serrano, 1975). The nutritional status of infants, mothers, and other family members is compromised by large family size, especially where resources are scarce (Maine, 1981). Thus, an effective family planning service—offering a wide range of contraceptive choices, including sterilization—can have a positive impact on infant health by reducing the incidence of high-order pregnancies and births to older women.

Health risks associated with female sterilization

Female sterilization compares very favourably with other contraceptive methods in terms of its safety. All contraceptives pose some health risks to users, although these risks are quite small in relation to those associated with pregnancy.

The specific health risks associated with female sterilization are limited mainly to complications occurring at the time of the surgical procedure or shortly thereafter. A detailed discussion of the side-effects and possible complications appears in Chapter 12. Studies from both developed and developing countries indicate that the mortality rate for female sterilization is less than 10 per 100 000.

History and current status

Female sterilization procedures were first performed in the late 1800s but did not become widely available until the 1930s, when the Pomeroy technique for ligating the tubes was introduced. Even then, and for several decades thereafter, most of these procedures were performed for medical or "eugenic" indications.

The 1960s brought an increasing interest in voluntary sterilization and the development of other modern birth control techniques. The introduction of new technology and simpler, safer, and more effective surgical techniques during the 1970s helped to bring the female sterilization procedure to its present position as the leading method of contraception worldwide.

Table 1 summarizes the available data on the use of female sterilization in 70 developing and developed countries or territories. Over 90 million women have been sterilized in these regions; the global figure is estimated to be about 140 million.

Table 1. Prevalence of female sterilization and number of women sterilized, for 70 countries or territories

Country or territory	Year	Prevalence[a] (%)	Estimated number of married women of reproductive age (in thousands)[b]	Estimated number of sterilized women (in thousands)[c]
Africa/Eastern Mediterranean				
Botswana	1984	1	85	0.9
Egypt	1988[d]	2	7 310	146.0
Ghana	1988[d]	1	2 164	21.6
Iraq	1974[e]	1	2 000	20.0
Jordan	1983	3	291[e]	8.7
Kenya (15–49)	1989[d]	5	3 279	163.9
Lesotho	1977	1	171	1.7
Liberia (15–49)	1986	1	342	3.4
Mauritius	1985	4	147	5.9
Morocco (15–49)	1987	2	3 235	64.7
South Africa	1976[e]	5	4 100[e]	205.0
Tunisia	1983	13	1 731[f]	225.0
Turkey	1983	1	7 304	73.0
Zimbabwe	1988[d]	2	1 323	26.5
Total				966.3
Asia				
Bangladesh	1985	8	17 596	1 407.7
China	1985	27	163 022	44 015.9
Fiji	1978[e]	17	100	17.0
Hong Kong	1977	19	505[e]	96.0
India	1982	11	123 407	13 577.8
Indonesia	1987	3	29 185	875.6
Republic of Korea	1985	32	5 982	1 914.2
Malaysia	1984	8	2 284	182.7
Nepal	1986	7	2 952	206.6
Pakistan	1985	2	14 471	289.4
Philippines	1986	10	8 108	810.8
Singapore	1983	22	354	77.9
Sri Lanka	1987	25	2 307	576.8
Thailand	1987	22	8 156	1 794.3
Total				65 842.7
Latin America/Caribbean				
Barbados	1981[e]	14	40[e]	5.6
Bolivia (15–49)	1989[d]	4	882	35.3
Brazil	1986	27	18 928	5 110.6

Table 1. (cont.)

Country or territory	Year	Prevalence[a] (%)	Estimated number of married women of reproductive age (in thousands)[b]	Estimated number of sterilized women (in thousands)[c]
Colombia (15–49)	1986	17	3 975	675.8
Costa Rica	1986	16	370	59.2
Cuba	1980[e]	16	1 700[e]	272.0
Dominican Republic (15–49)	1986	27	964	260.3
Ecuador (15–49)	1987	15	1 290	193.5
El Salvador	1988[g]	30	671	201.3
Guadeloupe	1976[e]	8	50[e]	4.0
Guatemala	1987	10	1 167	116.7
Guyana	1975	9	214	19.3
Haiti	1983	1	1 293[f]	12.9
Honduras	1984	12	540	64.8
Jamaica (15–49)	1983	11	568[h]	62.5
Martinique	1976[e]	9	50[e]	4.5
Mexico (15–49)	1987	19	11 544	2 193.4
Panama	1984	35	272	95.2
Paraguay	1987[g]	4	525	21.0
Peru (15–49)	1986	6	2 506	150.4
Puerto Rico	1982	40	400[e]	160.0
Venezuela	1977[e]	7	2 100[e]	147.0
Total				9 865.3
Developed countries				
Australia	1979[e]	22	2 400[e]	528.0
Austria	1982	1	1 882[f]	18.8
Belgium	1983	17	2 419[f]	411.2
Bulgaria	1976	1	1 700[e]	17.0
Canada	1984	31	4 353[f]	1 349.4
Czechoslovakia	1977	3	2 600[e]	78.0
Finland	1977	4	700[e]	28.0
France	1978	4	8 200[e]	328.0
Germany, Federal Republic of	1985	10	15 639[f]	1 563.9
Italy	1979	1	13 848[f]	138.5
Japan	1986	8	30 789[f]	2 463.1
Netherlands	1985	5	3 810[f]	190.5
New Zealand	1976	11	500[e]	55.0
Norway	1977	4	600[e]	24.0
Portugal (15–49)	1980	1	2 570[f]	25.7

Table 1. (cont.)

Country or territory	Year	Prevalence[a] (%)	Estimated number of married women of reproductive age (in thousands)[b]	Estimated number of sterilized women (in thousands)[c]
Spain	1985	4	9 342[f]	373.7
Sweden	1981	3	1 968[f]	59.0
Switzerland	1980	16	1 423[f]	227.7
United Kingdom	1983	14	13 354[f]	1 869.6
United States of America	1982	17	39 783[f]	6 763.1
Total				16 511.3
Overall total				93 185.6

[a] Prevalence rates represent the percentage of married women of reproductive age (15–44, unless noted otherwise). Except where noted, prevalence rates are from Mauldin & Segal, 1988.
[b] Except where noted, estimates are from Ross et al., 1988.
[c] Equal to the prevalence rate multiplied by the estimated number of married women of reproductive age.
[d] Data from Institute for Resource Development.
[e] Ross et al., 1985.
[f] UNFPA, 1985.
[g] Data from Centers for Disease Control.

Demand for female sterilization services is expected to increase in the future for a number of reasons, including the growing number of couples eligible for contraception due to increased urbanization and education, and a corresponding decrease in desired family size in many countries. It has been estimated that by the year 2010 the number of women undergoing female sterilization in developing countries, excluding China, will have increased by 109 million (Gillespie et al., 1988).

Factors affecting availability

Just as for any contraceptive method, the factors determining whether female sterilization is available in a community include the interest and commitment of health professionals, who in turn may be influenced by legal, political, religious, and other considerations. The accessibility and use of female sterilization services, on the other hand, depend more on the design of the service and the many factors affecting an individual client's decision to use a particular service. The factors related to availability are discussed below.

Laws and regulations

The legal status and means of delivering sterilization may be determined by statutory law, court decision, ministerial or other governmental regulation or decree, codes of medical ethics, or accepted practice. Service managers must be aware of the legal status of sterilization for their country or area, and how its delivery is regulated. Health authorities, medical associations, and legal authorities are often valuable sources for this kind of information.

Voluntary sterilization is legal in most jurisdictions. Some jurisdictions may allow the procedure only for medical indications, but health care staff generally have discretion to determine what constitutes a medical indication for sterilization. Similarly, some jurisdictions allow sterilization only for "social indications", but give providers discretion in determining what this actually constitutes. In other jurisdictions sterilization is considered legal even though no specific laws or regulations have made it so.

In a few countries the legal status of sterilization is unclear because laws against mutilation were once interpreted as prohibiting sterilization. However, where courts have considered the question in recent times, laws of this kind have been interpreted as not prohibiting the procedure.

Sterilization is illegal by statute, regulation, or decree in very few countries. The trend is to legalize the procedure. Between 1973 and 1983 at least 24 countries changed their laws and regulations to make voluntary sterilization legal.

Jurisdictions that allow sterilization, for whatever reason, often impose restrictions on how it is to be provided (see page 69 regarding informed consent). Some establish minimum standards that must be met in terms of the age of the client and the age, number, and sex of her living children, while others require the consent of the spouse. Such restrictions may have no legal basis. In that case, service managers should examine the restrictions to determine their effects on the accessibility of female sterilization.

More detailed information about laws and regulations affecting sterilization is available in the following references: Isaacs & Cook, 1984; Ross et al., 1985; and Ross et al., 1988.

Sociocultural and religious factors

Cultural patterns and traditions related to the role of women and to the importance of childbearing can influence the availability and acceptability of female sterilization. Certain beliefs and misinformation about the procedure that are prevalent among certain cultures or groups—for example, that those who undergo sterilization will be sterile when reincarnated, or that sterilization can make a woman weak and affect her sexuality—can discourage women from choosing this method. In such situations, services have a responsibility to provide accurate information and clarify misunderstandings about the nature of female sterilization, and to educate women and the community about the importance of women having control over their own fertility.

Religion may affect the availability of sterilization services. Opposition to sterilization by some religious leaders may encourage restrictive laws and policies or may influence public opinion so that health care staff hesitate to offer these services. Numerous studies have shown, however, that where sterilization is available, religious beliefs or practices have not affected requests for it (Philliber & Philliber, 1985). Followers of all the world's major religions have undergone sterilization. Indeed, service managers and staff may want to emphasize certain aspects of the service that religious leaders are likely to view favourably, such as the provision of sterilization for health reasons and medical indications.

Professional commitment

The involvement and leadership of health professionals (both clinicians and managerial personnel) are critical to the success of female sterilization services. Because they are respected members of the community, they can affect public policy and public acceptance. In addition, since health professionals formulate regulations and guidelines about client eligibility and the use of facilities, they can enhance or restrict access to female sterilization services. The importance of professional commitment and leadership cannot be overstated. Chapter 3 provides more information about the health care community and the categories and roles of professionals involved in female sterilization services.

Access and acceptance: the client's perspective

Where female sterilization services are available, their design and management significantly affect their accessibility, which in turn, influences their acceptability. To be successful, family planning services must aim to achieve client satisfaction. From the client's perspective, a number of features in the design of female sterilization services have an important bearing on satisfaction with them. These features are outlined in Table 2 and discussed in greater detail in subsequent chapters.

Advantages and disadvantages

There is no ideal contraceptive method suitable for all clients. Successful family planning services typically offer a wide range of methods in order to satisfy the requirements of as many clients as possible. Each method has advantages and disadvantages that must be considered in the design and management of services, and female sterilization is no different in this regard.

Comparison with other methods

If properly performed, female sterilization is a highly effective method of contraception, which compares very favourably with temporary methods. Inconvenience, side-effects, irregular supply, and forgetfulness can easily contribute to the failure of temporary methods. Clients must sustain a high level of motivation to use most temporary contraceptives. Likewise, clients require a very high degree of motivation to request and submit to female sterilization surgery, and its attendant risks. However, in contrast to users of temporary methods, a woman who has undergone a successful sterilization does not subsequently need to practise family planning.

Failure rates for various contraceptive methods—the percentage of clients who become pregnant during the first year of using a particular method—are presented in Table 3, which is based on data from the United States of America. Two rates are

Table 2. Selected service design features influencing the accessibility and provision of female sterilization

Design feature	Purpose	Additional information
Information sources	To provide accurate information at the community level that corrects erroneous information, allays fears, and informs women where services are available through channels such as word of mouth, printed materials, group meetings, and mass media.	Chapter 6
Client referral	To guide interested clients to clinics through community-based networks such as women's groups, family planning services, and the local medical community.	Page 31 Chapter 6
Number and location of service sites	To ensure convenience and access through the establishment of services that are strategically located and sufficient in number.	Chapters 3–4
Client eligibility criteria, screening procedures, counselling, and informed consent	To ensure client satisfaction through attention to the assurance of free and informed choice.	Chapter 7
Standards for interacting with clients	To enhance the acceptability and reputation of the service by treating all clients with respect and concern.	Page 38
Medical service standards	To ensure effectiveness and minimize complications and discomfort through strict application of medical standards and attention to the assurance of medical safety.	Chapters 8–12
Cost to client	To enhance access to services by establishing affordable fee structures, if clients are to be charged.	Chapter 1, Chapter 5
Data collection, monitoring and service evaluation	To detect and correct problems and service deficiencies through well-maintained and properly used record-keeping and monitoring systems.	Chapter 17

Table 3. Failure rates of various contraceptive methods in the United States of America

Method	First year failure rates (%)	
	Lowest expected	Typical
Chance	89	89
Spermicides	3	21
Periodic abstinence		20
Ovulation method	8	
Symptothermal	6	
Calendar	10	
Postovulation	2	
Withdrawal	4	18
Cap, with spermicidal cream or jelly	5	18
Sponge	5 (nulliparous) >8 (parous)	18 (nulliparous) >28 (parous)
Diaphragm, with spermicidal cream or jelly	3	18
Condom, without spermicide	2	12
IUD		6
medicated	1	
non-medicated	2	
Pill		3
combined	0.1	
progestogen only	0.5	
Injectable progestogen		
depot medroxyprogesterone acetate	0.3	0.3
norethisterone enantate	0.4	0.4
Implants		
capsules	0.3	0.3
rods	0.2	0.2
Female sterilization	0.2	0.4
Male sterilization	0.1	0.15

Source: Trussell & Kost, 1987. Used by permission.

given for each method: the lowest expected rate, which is an estimate of the proportion of couples who will experience an accidental pregnancy even if they use the method correctly and consistently; and the typical effectiveness rate, which takes into account that methods are not always perfectly delivered by service providers or perfectly used by couples. It can be seen that methods that depend on a service provider for their delivery or application, including sterilization, implants, injectables, and intrauterine devices, are generally more effective than those that rely more on the active and conscious involvement of the user. In fact, since the data on which these rates are based have not been adjusted for under-reporting of abortion, the failure rates for client-dependent methods may be even higher (Jones & Forrest, 1989).

Cost

Although the cost of sterilization is usually high, it does not carry recurring costs, either to the client or the service, as do temporary methods. Thus, when its cost is amortized—i.e., spread out over the remaining years of a couple's reproductive capacity—the cost of a year's protection using sterilization compares very favourably with that of other contraceptive methods. However, costs may vary with different sterilization procedures according to the equipment, training, anaesthesia, and expendable supplies required. Costs may also differ according to the mode of service delivery (Huber & Harvey, 1989). (See Chapter 5 for further details.)

Eligibility

Since female sterilization is intended to be permanent, it should be provided only to individuals who have definitely decided to have no more children. Services should present it as one of many contraceptive options, all of which should either be readily available at the same site or be available through referral at a nearby outlet. Staff must carefully screen and counsel potential clients about all methods so that clients can give consent based on full information and free choice. Such factors as the client's age, her health and mental status, and the ages and number of her children must be taken into consideration. However, staff should not use these factors arbitrarily to deny access to sterilization for those who have made a free and informed choice of this method (see Chapter 7).

2. Female sterilization techniques and service choices

Minilaparotomy and laparoscopy have become the preferred procedures for female sterilization, since they are simple, safe, and inexpensive, and can be made available in a variety of settings. They enable health care providers to offer female sterilization on an outpatient basis, and as either a postpartum or an interval procedure.

Techniques

The fundamental objective of female sterilization—to block the fallopian tubes so preventing fertilization—may be achieved by various techniques, all of which must be evaluated for their relative safety, effectiveness, and service compatibility.

However, some techniques are more appropriate for use with certain surgical approaches than with others, and both of these factors are affected by the timing of the procedure (see Table 4). More detailed discussion of the surgical technique is provided in Chapter 10.

Timing of female sterilization

Female sterilization may be performed throughout most of a woman's reproductive life. It may be done shortly after a vaginal delivery, in conjunction with a caesarean section, immediately following a nonseptic abortion, or during a period when the woman has not recently been pregnant. Usually sterilization is not performed when the woman is pregnant or during days 8–41 following delivery, when the surgery may be more difficult. However, some services reportedly perform minilaparotomies during this later postpartum period without higher complication rates.

The following definitions are used throughout these guidelines to describe the timing of sterilization:

Table 4. Timing, surgical approach, and occlusive techniques for female sterilization

Timing	Surgical approach	Occlusive technique: Recommended/ preferred	Occlusive technique: Acceptable alternatives[a]
Interval	Minilaparotomy	Pomeroy Parkland	Silicone band Filshie clip Spring clip
	Laparoscopy	Silicone band Filshie clip Spring clip	Electro-coagulation[b]
	Laparotomy[c]	Pomeroy Parkland	Silicone band Filshie clip Spring clip
Postpartum	Minilaparotomy	Pomeroy Parkland	Filshie clip
	Laparotomy (caesarean section)	Pomeroy Parkland Irving	Filshie clip
Postabortion	Minilaparotomy	Pomeroy Parkland	Silicone band Filshie clip Spring clip
	Laparoscopy	Silicone band Filshie clip	Spring clip

[a] These are generally acceptable alternatives, although "recommended/preferred" methods are considered better for routine use in terms of cost, simplicity, or associated risks.

[b] Many countries (including the United States of America and Canada) do not consider electrocoagulation an acceptable alternative for routine use.

[c] Laparotomy may be done in cases where other approaches are not appropriate because of factors such as obesity and pelvic scarring.

- *Postpartum* refers to sterilizations performed at the same time as caesarean section or within 41 days after vaginal delivery. The latter are usually performed during the first 48 hours after delivery or, with special care, during days 3–7 after delivery; procedures are generally not performed on days 8–41.
- *Postabortion* refers to sterilizations performed immediately following nonseptic induced or spontaneous termination of pregnancy.

- *Interval* refers to sterilizations performed 6 weeks (42 days) or more after the last delivery.

In addition, the term "pregnancy-related sterilization" is used to refer to both postpartum and postabortion sterilization procedures.

Variations in surgical approach

Abdominal approaches. Of the three possible approaches to the fallopian tubes—abdominal, vaginal, and transcervical—the abdominal approaches are used most commonly. Laparotomy, minilaparotomy, and laparoscopy are included in this category. Conventional laparotomy (involving an abdominal incision exceeding 5 cm) usually requires hospitalization, the use of general or regional anaesthesia, and a relatively long recovery period. This approach poses a greater risk of complications than the other abdominal approaches; therefore, it is infrequently used except for obese women, in complicated and emergency cases, or when sterilization is performed in conjunction with caesarean section.

Minilaparotomy is an adaptation of conventional laparotomy, involving a smaller abdominal incision (3–4 cm), which means that it can be performed as an outpatient procedure using local anaesthesia and light sedation.[1] For both laparotomy and minilaparotomy, the surgeon usually lifts the fallopian tubes out of the abdomen to occlude them. Both of these approaches can be used in the interval period, postabortion, and up to one week after delivery.

Laparoscopy uses an endoscopic, or optical, instrument (the laparoscope), which is inserted into the abdomen, allowing the operator to visualize and occlude the fallopian tubes within the abdomen. While laparoscopy has proved to be almost as safe and reliable as minilaparotomy and takes somewhat less time, it is a more sophisticated procedure and is best performed by gynaecologists or other surgical specialists (Mumford et al.,

---

[1] In a previous WHO publication, *Surgery at the district hospital: obstetrics, gynaecology, orthopaedics, and traumatology* (Cook et al., 1991), it is stated that while local anaesthesia with light sedation is sufficient for minilaparotomy procedures, general or regional anaesthesia is preferred. However, it should be borne in mind that the present guidelines are for surgeons carrying out female sterilization in the field, where facilities and equipment may be limited. For surgeons who are skilled in female sterilization procedures, local anaesthesia with light sedation is considered to be adequate.

1980). This approach should not be used in the postpartum period or postabortion when gestation is greater than 12 weeks. Distinctions between laparoscopy and minilaparotomy are discussed further on pages 21, and 100–105.

Vaginal approaches include colpotomy, which uses direct vision and standard surgical instruments, and culdoscopy, which employs an endoscopic instrument to reach the fallopian tubes through the posterior wall of the vagina. These approaches were popular in the early 1970s, as they could be performed quickly using local anaesthesia, but studies demonstrating relatively high rates of infection, pain, surgical accidents, and failure have led to their virtual elimination (Cummins, 1976; WHO Task Force on Female Sterilization, 1982c). Vaginal approaches are also discussed on page 106.

Transcervical approaches employ either the hysteroscope (a specialized endoscope) or blind transcervical manipulation (which depends on the operator's sense of touch) to reach the fallopian tubes through the cervix and uterus. These approaches are still considered experimental and have generally been less effective than standard techniques (Zatuchni et al., 1983). They are discussed further on page 106.

Variations in methods of tubal occlusion

A number of techniques of tubal occlusion have been developed in an attempt to improve effectiveness, reliability, and safety; to make the procedure quicker and easier for the surgeon; to reduce client discomfort; and to minimize tubal damage. However, only a few techniques are commonly used today, and these can be grouped into four categories: ligation and division, mechanical methods, electrical methods, and other methods. Examples of recommended and commonly used occlusive methods are illustrated in Fig. 2; their respective advantages and disadvantages are presented in Table 5.

Ligation and division methods involve tying each fallopian tube with suture material (ligation), cutting it (division), and, in some cases, removing a section of the tube (resection). These techniques must be used in conjunction with the minilaparotomy approach; they cannot be used in combination with laparoscopy. The Pomeroy procedure, which involves tying a loop of each tube with absorbable suture (catgut) and cutting off the knuckle

Fig. 2. Selected occlusive techniques for female sterilization

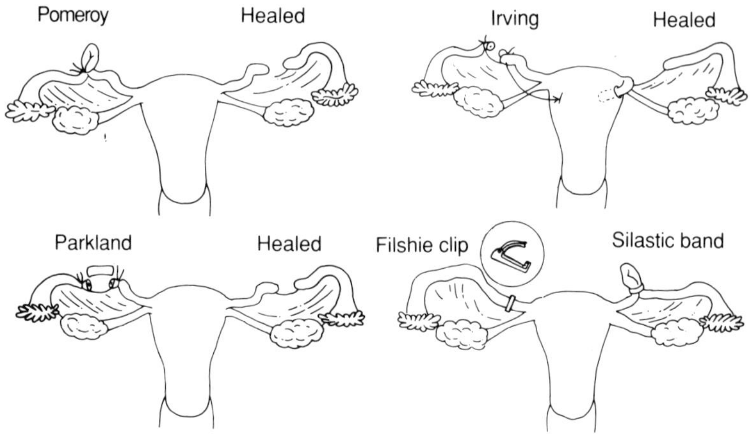

Adapted from Hatcher et al., 1988. Used by permission.

of the loop near the tie, is the most commonly used method of ligation and resection. The Parkland technique is another effective method, which involves tying the tube at two points and removing the small intervening segment.

Two ligation and division techniques that were used previously are the Uchida and the Irving techniques. Both are very effective, but require large incisions (the Irving has been done during caesarean section) and, because of their more complicated nature, take a relatively long time to perform.

Other ligation methods rarely used today are fimbriectomy (Kroener), salpingectomy, and the Madlener and Aldrich techniques.

Mechanical methods are now the preferred means of occlusion used with laparoscopy. They involve placing a device, such as a small band or ring made of silicone rubber, to close and seal each fallopian tube. The band, which is effective, safe, and inexpensive, requires a special attachment to the laparoscope for application.

Clips represent a second group of mechanical occlusive devices, which were developed primarily for use with a laparoscope; however, they may also be used with minilaparotomy. The Filshie clip, which is a hinged titanium device lined with silicone rubber, and the spring-loaded Hulka or Wolf clip are the most widely used clips. One advantage of clips is that they destroy

Table 5. Advantages and disadvantages of selected occlusive techniques for female sterilization

Technique	Advantages	Disadvantages
Ligation and division		
Pomeroy Parkland	Effective; suitable for postpartum and interval cases; low rate of complications; simple; specialist surgeon not needed; inexpensive	Cannot be used with laparoscopy
Irving	Highly effective, can be done during caesarean section	More difficult to perform than Pomeroy and Parkland; requires more time, and may cause more bleeding during surgery; requires laparotomy; destroys more tubal tissue
Mechanical		
Silicone band Filshie clip Spring clip	Destroy less tubal tissue than ligation; fast; suitable for interval cases using laparoscopy in high-volume settings	Usually applied by laparoscopy, which requires specialist surgeon and laparoscopy training; more expensive than ligation and division; rates of failures and complications can increase if training is inadequate or skills not maintained; less suitable for postpartum use than Parkland and Pomeroy
Electrical		
Electro-coagulation	Can be performed via laparoscopy; fast; may cause less post-operative pain than mechanical techniques	Usually destroys more tubal tissue; requires specialist surgeon and laparoscopy training; rates of failures and complications can increase if training inadequate or skills are not maintained; associated with serious complications (internal burns); ectopic pregnancies higher than with mechanical techniques; not officially approved or endorsed for general use by many countries

considerably less tubal tissue than all other techniques of occlusion, thus rendering reversal surgery, if attempted, technically simpler (see page 124). Disadvantages of clips include their high cost relative to bands and the need for specialist training to use them.

Electrical methods (electrocoagulation, fulguration, diathermy) are usually used with a laparoscope to coagulate (or cauterize) and block the fallopian tubes. While generally effective, electrical methods have been associated with burns to the bowel, bladder, and abdominal wall, as well as with a higher risk of later ectopic pregnancy than ligation and mechanical methods (Whong, 1987; WFHAAVSC, 1988).

Other methods of occlusion, which are experimental and have not yet been proved effective and applicable for widespread use, include insertion of removable plugs into the fallopian tubes and the instillation of chemical agents that scar the tubes.

Service considerations: postpartum and interval female sterilization

From the service perspective, the advantages of offering both postpartum and interval sterilization are significant. If services are made readily available, this improves their accessibility, which means that they are more likely to be accepted. Postpartum sterilization services are an integral part of complete maternity care. The convenience of postpartum services means fewer missed appointments, and these services also integrate more easily within the health care system, since they may use existing facilities (hospitals and maternity centres) and personnel, which in turn helps to keep costs low and improves the prospects for long-term continuation of services.

From the surgical perspective, minilaparotomy performed within 48 hours after vaginal delivery is easier than and as safe and effective as interval minilaparotomy and laparoscopy (Indian Council of Medical Research, 1982; WHO Task Force on Female Sterilization, 1982a). Because of the enlargement of the uterus postpartum, the fallopian tubes are nearer the incision, and can be reached easily during the first 48 hours after delivery. However, from day 3 to day 7 after delivery, more care is required, since the uterus becomes less accessible as it contracts and bacteria may have entered the tubes. Prophylactic antibiotics may be given during this period and when minilaparotomy is performed on days 8–41.

From the client's perspective, postpartum sterilization eliminates the need for a second visit to a hospital or clinic, and the normal hospital stay required for delivery need not be prolonged. Furthermore, postpartum minilaparotomy requires less instrumentation and causes less discomfort to the client than interval sterilization; lighter sedation and analgesia may often be used (see page 100).

The specific circumstances of every country must determine the relative balance and availability of both interval and postpartum sterilization services. Countries where the maternal health care infrastructure is not well developed and where most deliveries take place at home may tend to rely more on interval than on postpartum services.

Elsewhere, government policies may influence the balance of postpartum and interval services. In some Latin American countries, for example, governments do not actively support sterilization services. As a result, these services are provided by non-governmental family planning associations, which do not usually attend deliveries and can offer only interval sterilizations.

In countries such as Brazil (where sterilization is the most popular method of contraception), sterilization procedures are not reimbursed by the government, unless performed for certain medical conditions. A large proportion of these procedures have been performed in conjunction with caesarean section deliveries, and many observers link this to the restrictive policy. By contrast, in countries where the government actively supports sterilization services and where the infrastructure permits, both interval and postpartum sterilization services are widely available; Mexico and Thailand are examples.

The service implications for setting up postpartum or interval services are summarized in Table 6.

Service considerations: minilaparotomy and laparoscopy

In large-scale studies, minilaparotomy and laparoscopy have proved to be almost equally safe and effective (McCann, 1978; Mumford et al., 1980; Ross et al., 1985; WHO Task Force on Female Sterilization, 1982b), and debate continues about which is the more appropriate approach for use in national and

Table 6. Comparison of postpartum and interval female sterilization

Consideration	Postpartum	Interval
Information and education (see Chapter 6)	Should be provided during antenatal visits to clinics, or during home visits by midwives or other field-workers.	May be provided at any time through a variety of interpersonal and mass media communications channels.
Counselling and informed consent (see Chapter 7)	Preferably during antenatal period, although possible after delivery if client is well recovered and lucid. Must *not* be done during labour, or when the woman is experiencing stress.	No general problems with timing prior to sterilization.
Service-delivery channels (see Chapter 3)	Normally restricted to permanent, multipurpose settings (those hospitals and maternity centres attending deliveries).	May be done in multipurpose hospitals, free-standing clinics, or via temporary, mobile services.
Instruments and equipment (see Chapter 16)	Requires simple, standard instruments, fewer than required for interval minilaparotomy or laparoscopy.	Minilaparotomy requires uterine manipulator and pelvic examination equipment; laparoscopy requires sophisticated endoscopic systems.
Costs and sustainability (see Chapter 5)	Generally less costly than interval sterilization because requires less anaesthesia, no additional hospitalization, and less equipment, and is easily integrated with existing staff and facilities, therefore may be more sustainable.	May be more costly, depending on technique used, type of setting, and type of service-delivery channel.
Surgical skills and expertise	Generally easier to perform, since postpartum uterus brings tubes closer to abdominal wall. Good for training in minilaparotomy; laparoscopy cannot be performed at this time.	Can be more difficult, requiring more manipulation of uterus to bring tubes to the incision site. A feasible time to perform laparoscopy.

large-scale services (Chaturachinda, 1976; Liskin et al., 1985; McCann, 1978).

The techniques of minilaparotomy and laparoscopy are compared in Table 7. This comparison suggests that minilaparotomy is the more appropriate method for use in most national or large-scale services, since it requires simple, inexpensive, easily maintained equipment and may be performed by any doctor who has some surgical experience, following a period of training. Furthermore, minilaparotomy is the indicated approach for postpartum services. As the costs associated with starting and maintaining minilaparotomy services are less than those for laparoscopy, these services are easier for health care systems to sustain.

On the other hand, laparoscopy has proven advantages for use in tertiary-level urban facilities, which have a concentration of skilled surgeons and a sufficient case-load to maintain specialized surgical skills. The volume of services also helps to offset the costs of purchasing and maintaining the more expensive laparoscopy equipment. All laparoscopists should have the skills and equipment to perform minilaparotomy or laparotomy in the event of surgical difficulty, electrical failure, or other emergencies.

In summary, each facility must determine which method of sterilization is most appropriate for its circumstances and context. In many settings, minilaparotomy offers the best option for safely extending services to the largest number of clients. In settings with well-developed health infrastructures, which have adequate case-loads for surgeons to maintain skills, access to repair and maintenance services, and the ability to absorb the costs of repair and maintenance, laparoscopy may be the technique of choice. In many countries, a combination of minilaparotomy, offered extensively in basic facilities and in rural areas, with laparoscopy, provided in a few high-volume urban centres, may be most effective.

Conclusions and recommendations

The technique used for female sterilization should ideally:

- be reliably effective and associated with very low failure rates;
- be relatively simple and thereby usable by the lowest appropriate category of personnel trained to perform

Table 7. Comparison of minilaparotomy and laparoscopy for female sterilization

	Minilaparotomy	Laparoscopy
Instruments and equipment (see Chapter 16)	Requires a few inexpensive, standard surgical instruments.	Requires delicate, sophisticated, and expensive endoscopic equipment, which needs to be maintained.
Surgical skills and expertise (see Chapter 3)	Can be performed by any doctor with basic surgical ability and skills, after training in the technique.	Restricted to specially trained surgeons and gynaecologists. Requires regular practice to maintain skills.
Setting (see Chapter 15)	May be performed in maternity centres and basic health facilities with surgical capacity.	Anaesthetist required. Back-up facilities advisable.
Time	Usually performed in 10–20 minutes.	Performed in 5–15 minutes. Useful for services with large daily case-loads.
Contraindications (see Chapter 8)	Difficult to use for obese women (especially for interval procedures) and those with pelvic scarring and adhesions. (See also page 79.)	Not recommended for post-partum use or for women with previous lower abdominal surgery or pelvic infections.
Complications (see Chapter 12)	Relatively low complication rate. Risks of bowel and bladder injuries, uterine perforation. Slightly higher rate of wound infection than with laparoscopy. Injury to mesosalpinx may require additional surgery or laparotomy.	Low complication rate. Slight risk of life-threatening vascular injury, bowel injury and insufflation accidents. Severing the tube or injury to mesosalpinx may require laparotomy.
Side-effects (see Chapter 12)	Short-term abdominal pain may occur.	Postoperative chest and shoulder pain resulting from abdominal insufflation.
Effectiveness (see Chapter 13)	Highly effective; failure rates <1% after 12 months for most occlusive techniques.	Highly effective; failure rates <1% after 12 months for most occlusive techniques.

Sources: Adapted from Chaturachinda, 1976, and Liskin et al., 1985.

surgery, and in the largest possible number of health care facilities;
- be safe, posing minimal risks of serious complications;
- be relatively pain-free when performed under local anaesthesia, and as comfortable as possible for the client;
- affect only fertility, and no other physiological functions;
- be inexpensive;
- be suitable for application on an outpatient basis, if possible, or when following delivery, without the need for added hospitalization; and
- cause minimum tubal damage, thus improving the chances of successful reversal.

Only a small number of the possible female sterilization techniques meet all or even most of the above criteria. However, bearing in mind these criteria and the foregoing discussion, the following recommendations can be made for planners and managers of family planning services:

- To increase the availability and use of services, both pregnancy-related and interval female sterilization should be readily available.
- For most developing countries, minilaparotomy is the technique that permits the safest and most cost-effective service to be offered to the largest number of potential clients, while at the same time making the best use of existing facilities and personnel.
- Laparoscopy can be used safely and relatively cost-effectively in areas that have a well-developed health care system. It should be performed by trained specialists in institutions where the case-load is sufficient for them to maintain their skills. Laparoscopy services must also have the resources (skills and equipment) to perform minilaparotomy or laparotomy when necessary and to maintain and repair the sophisticated equipment.
- Services should promote occlusive techniques that minimize damage to the fallopian tubes. The tubal clip method inflicts the least damage but is significantly more expensive than other techniques. Ligation and resection techniques and use of silicone bands are cheaper and, when performed carefully, yield an acceptable potential for reversal.
- Although sterilization can be carried out during caesarean section and is also accomplished by hysterectomy (see page 107), these approaches involve major surgery and

should never be used for the primary objective of achieving sterilization.

- The following procedures are *not recommended* for general use in female sterilization services because of their probable higher rates of failure or complications (see pages 101 and 106):

  —postpartum laparoscopy
  —vaginal approaches (colpotomy, culdoscopy)
  —fimbriectomy (Kroener)
  —salpingectomy
  —all currently available transcervical (mainly experimental) approaches.

3. Female sterilization and the health care system

Female sterilization services should be fully linked with the existing public and private health care systems, particularly the maternity and family planning services. Selecting the appropriate service-delivery channels and personnel to provide female sterilization is crucial for the safety, acceptability, and ease of access of these services. Maximum appropriate use should be made of existing facilities, service-delivery opportunities, and suitably qualified personnel, and training opportunities should be expanded to increase the number of personnel involved. Systems for client referral and follow-up should also be established within the existing health care structure.

Service-delivery channels

Because female sterilization is a surgical procedure, there are limitations as to where and how it can be provided. The simplicity of the procedure, however, makes it possible to deliver these services closer to the community than might be expected. While a fully equipped hospital is not required, the facilities should include a waiting room/reception area, an examination room, access to laboratory services, and a clean surgical area isolated from the outside and from clinic traffic (see Chapter 15).

Although most female sterilizations are performed in permanent sites, it is possible for the procedure to be carried out by mobile surgical teams. These teams usually operate by making periodic visits to existing permanent health facilities that have no staff trained to perform female sterilization. Where health facilities are not available, teams may operate in other suitably adapted settings, such as schools or community buildings. In a few services, mobile teams use specially equipped vehicles, in which the operation can be performed, to travel to underserved locations.

Several countries—including Colombia, Guatemala, India, Nepal, and the Philippines—have successfully used mobile teams to offer female sterilization services to rural, remote, or underserved communities. However, mobile teams are usually costly, requiring more resources (e.g., personnel) than services provided in permanent facilities (Jezowski & Ellis, 1987; McBride et al., 1987). Service providers must devote extra attention to quality assurance because it may be more difficult to maintain cleanliness and asepsis, to screen and counsel clients, and to provide postoperative follow-up and treatment of complications in a mobile setting (see page 31). Furthermore, because mobile teams may need to travel long distances, and may work long hours under difficult and unfamiliar conditions, they must take extra care to avoid mistakes.[1] The mobile teams should be staffed with the most proficient and experienced personnel available, who must be experts at preventing problems and at immediately recognizing and managing any that do occur. These personnel must be given the opportunity to maintain their surgical skills through regular practice.

Because extra resources are required for mobile services, fewer funds may be available to train personnel and equip permanent facilities in the areas served by mobile teams. When the demand for sterilization grows to a suitable level in these areas, managers should consider reallocating resources to establish permanent services. Each country and community must study its own conditions, resources, and priorities to determine whether mobile teams are compatible with health needs and objectives in the area. In most situations, use of mobile teams should be viewed as a short-term measure to serve an area until either the demand for services or the availability of trained personnel and improved infrastructure permit the establishment of female sterilization services on a permanent basis (Jezowski & Ellis, 1987).

Integrated versus vertical (specialized) services

Integrating female sterilization services with other health care services has the advantage of making use of existing personnel,

---

[1] See *Safe and voluntary surgical contraception*, appendix A, published by the World Federation of Health Agencies for the Advancement of Voluntary Surgical Contraception, 1988, for quality assurance guidelines relating to the establishment and management of mobile voluntary sterilization services.

facilities, and other material resources. In addition, when sterilization is offered along with other family health services, its importance as a means of protecting health by reducing maternal morbidity and mortality is reinforced. A potential disadvantage of integration is that female sterilization services may be accorded lower priority by staff occupied with curative and emergency services.

Female sterilization services delivered in specialized outpatient centres may be more likely to sustain a high level of performance over an extended period of time. Resources, such as space, staff, and equipment, that are specifically allocated for female sterilization are less likely to be diverted for other purposes. In such settings, the surgical team becomes expert, and services can be offered efficiently and safely. However, unless the case-load is adequate, specialized services may not be economically viable. Another disadvantage is that specialized services may place undue emphasis on the numbers of procedures performed, which may result in inadequate attention being given to ensuring that clients make voluntary informed decisions.

Personnel requirements

The provision of female sterilization services requires a team effort. The number of personnel, their skills, and their training depend on the setting and situation in which the procedure is being performed, the case-load, and the surgical and anaesthetic techniques used. The team members are responsible for performing the following activities:

- Registering clients and maintaining records
- Providing information and education
- Counselling clients and obtaining informed consent
- Examining clients
- Performing laboratory tests
- Preparing and maintaining the operating theatre, equipment, and supplies
- Administering anaesthesia and performing surgery
- Providing postoperative monitoring and care
- Following up clients and conducting follow-up examinations
- Cleaning and maintaining the facility

The minimum staff requirement for the simplest procedure (a minilaparotomy using local anaesthesia) is a team comprising a surgeon, a surgical assistant, and a theatre attendant. In clinics with a small case-load, this team should be able to perform all the essential duties; however, more staff may be required as the case-load increases.

All staff members should receive precise, written job descriptions so that they are fully aware of the tasks they are expected to perform. Selected tasks, such as carrying out laboratory tests, and cleaning and maintaining the facility, may be contracted out.

Any medical doctor who has some surgical experience, preferably in abdominal surgery, can be trained to perform minilaparotomy. In situations where the number of doctors is not sufficient to meet the demand for female sterilization, nurses or paramedical staff have been trained to perform minilaparotomy under the supervision of a qualified doctor. It has been shown, for example, in Bangladesh and Thailand, that trained paramedical personnel may perform minilaparotomies as safely as doctors (Chowdhury & Chowdhury, 1975; Satyapan, 1983).

Compared with minilaparotomy, laparoscopy requires more staff and more highly skilled and experienced surgeons. Because laparoscopy equipment is technically complex and requires special handling, at least one staff member must receive special training in equipment maintenance. Furthermore, the physicians trained in laparoscopy should be fully competent obstetrician-gynaecologists, general surgeons, doctors with three years of training in obstetrics and gynaecology, or other medical doctors with a minimum of three years' experience in abdominal and pelvic surgery.

An anaesthetist must be present whenever general or regional anaesthesia is used for female sterilization. The anaesthetist, who may not necessarily be a medical doctor, should be available during laparoscopy in case serious complications arise that require more extensive surgery.

Training needs

The personnel requirements outlined above indicate that various training activities are required to ensure a high-quality female sterilization service. Service managers must make decisions about the design, location, and funding of training for the various tasks performed by the female sterilization team. When services are being introduced in a country or locality, surgical training may take place on specialized courses in another country, or in a training centre or teaching hospital within the country.

Training may then be expanded through the provision of additional training sites or through second-generation, on-site training by the initial group trained. The non-surgical tasks also require special training; these include administration of anaesthetic, maintenance of laparoscopy equipment, and counselling (see page 61 and Chapter 17).

At some stage, the service manager must determine the most cost-effective means of expanding training to meet growing demand for female sterilization. This may require coordination with national medical education authorities to ensure that training in various aspects of female sterilization is incorporated in the medical and paramedical training curricula. Ideally, surgical training should be carried out in teams of doctors and surgical assistants, since this method gives each member of the team the opportunity to learn the entire scope of the procedure, and encourages a team approach to service delivery.

Important links: client referrals and postoperative follow-up

Liaison with other health services to announce the availability of female sterilization is one means of informing the community about services and ensuring referrals. This is especially important during the early stages of a female sterilization service, before other means of referral, such as word of mouth and extensive informational campaigns, are in place. Other health providers can become important community supporters of female sterilization services if clients they refer are satisfied with the services received. They can also carry out follow-up examinations for clients who live closer to them than to the sterilization service site.

Special arrangements must be made for follow-up of women who are sterilized by a mobile surgical team that does not provide follow-up, or who find it difficult to return to the service site. If mobile teams are used, local doctors or community health personnel should be specially trained to conduct follow-up examinations. Paramedical staff must be trained to identify problems, to treat minor ones, and to refer clients to the nearest health centre when serious complications arise. Clients must be instructed to seek assistance if they encounter postoperative problems. (Postoperative care and instructions are discussed in more detail on page 71 and in Chapter 11.)

Staff of the female sterilization service must always be prepared to refer clients to higher levels of the health system when it is appropriate to do so. In the event of rare, life-threatening complications, the client may need to be transferred to another facility that is better equipped to handle the situation. If unrelated medical problems are discovered during the preoperative screening and examination, or if the client decides in favour of a method of contraception that is not available at the service site, the staff must be prepared to treat or refer the client. Occasionally, screening and counselling may identify psychological problems that require referral for further counselling or treatment.

4. Organizing and managing female sterilization services

The service manager's mandate

It is the responsibility of managers of sterilization services to make available safe, voluntary sterilization services to the largest possible number of potential users, and to do so using methods that are affordable and sustainable over the long term.

At the same time, managers must ensure that sterilization is provided under conditions that minimize the risks associated with elective surgery. Since sterilization directly and permanently ends reproduction, clients requesting this service must be given full information about its intended effects and consequences. Managers must ensure that services are offered without inducement or coercion, and that meticulous attention is given to medical safety.

Fig. 3 lists six principles that embody the responsibilities and challenges of managers of sterilization services. Of these, the first

Fig. 3. Principles for managers of sterilization services

Primary principles

Ensure that all clients make voluntary, fully informed, and well-considered decisions.

Ensure the medical safety and effectiveness of all clinical and surgical procedures.

Other principles

Establish services that are responsive to the needs, preferences, and behaviour of clients and the community.

Make services widely available and easily accessible to all potential clients.

Plan and manage services to ensure their efficiency and cost-effectiveness.

Strive for long-term viability and sustainability of services.

Table 8. Checklist for planning and organizing female sterilization services

	Activity	Additional information
1.	Survey community, identify potential obstacles.	Page 35
2.	Investigate laws, legal issues, regulations; obtain licences and other approvals.	Page 8
3.	Estimate potential case-load.	Page 36
4.	Develop budget; arrange financing.	Chapter 5
5.	Develop information and education programme.	Chapter 6
6.	Establish clinic facilities; select, prepare, and renovate site.	Page 131
7.	Arrange for supplies, equipment, and services:	Chapters 15 and 16
	(a) Procure equipment, instruments, medicines, and supplies.	
	(b) Establish storage and inventory systems.	
	(c) Establish procedures for sterilizing equipment and supplies.	
8.	Establish essential policies:	
	(a) Client-selection criteria.	Chapter 8
	(b) Procedures regarding free and informed decision-making, counselling, and informed consent.	Chapter 7
	(c) Medical/surgical protocols and service standards.	Chapters 8–12
9.	Develop and print record forms, information materials, and other documents:	
	(a) Medical history/client record form.	Page 77, Annex 5
	(b) Informed-consent form.	Page 69, Fig. 5.
	(c) Preoperative and postoperative instructions.	Page 71, Annex 2
	(d) Client brochures and other information materials.	Pages 49 and 54
10.	Staff the programme:	
	(a) Determine staff requirements, develop job descriptions.	Page 29
	(b) Recruitment and selection.	Page 29
	(c) Training.	Chapter 17, Page 29
11.	Establish client-flow system and procedures:	
	(a) Reception, intake, and registration.	Chapters 8 and 15
	(b) Record of patient history.	Page 77, Annex 5
	(c) Clinic-based information activities.	Page 55
	(d) Client counselling.	Page 61
	(e) Informed consent.	Pages 69 and 82
	(f) Physical examination and medical screening, including laboratory tests.	Pages 77 and 81
	(g) Referral for medical or psychological indications or for temporary contraception.	Pages 73 and 77

Table 8. (cont.)

	Activity	Additional information
	(h) Preoperative preparation.	Pages 71 and 82, Annex 2
	(i) Surgical procedure.	Chapters 9 and 10
	(j) Complications management and emergency treatment procedures.	Chapter 12
	(k) Postoperative monitoring.	Page 108
	(l) Postoperative instructions and discharge.	Page 71, Chapter 11, Annex 2
	(m) Follow-up procedures.	Page 109
12.	Other:	
	(a) Financial accounting procedures.	Chapter 5
	(b) Data collection and service statistics.	Page 160
	(c) Monitoring and evaluation.	Chapter 18

two are the most important, since they address the fundamental requirements that must be met if high-quality services are to be provided. These are that *managers must ensure that clients are fully informed and able to make a well-considered decision*, and that *services are of the highest possible medical quality*. The remaining principles are concerned with ensuring that these high-quality services are well utilized and successful.

Starting a new service

Systematic and thoughtful planning will result in services that are well attended, function smoothly, and satisfy clients. Table 8 provides a checklist for planning sterilization services. The table also indicates where additional information on each of these activities is available in these guidelines.

Assessing the local community situation

Before introducing female sterilization services, managers must consider the environment or community in which the services are to be located. Political, cultural, and religious obstacles must be identified and taken into account. Local laws and regulations, guidelines for medical practices, and codes of ethics should be studied to determine how they will affect services, and the necessary permits and licences must be obtained. (See also page 8.)

Managers should also investigate the level of community knowledge and practice of family planning, and the availability of other family planning services. Existing data, group discussions, and community surveys can help identify areas of misinformation about sterilization so that relevant changes can be made to the information and counselling components of the service. In addition, in this preliminary community survey, local medical and health professionals should be interviewed to determine their attitudes about and willingness to collaborate in the provision of female sterilization services.

Estimating the potential case-load

Given a particular population, the service manager will require an estimate of the potential demand for female sterilization in a given period of time. This estimate will be important in determining the facilities, staff, and other resources needed. The actual number of clients requesting services will be influenced by such variables as the cultural acceptability of sterilization, the design and accessibility of services, the existence of similar services in the community, and the impact of information and education.

Estimating potential demand is more an art than a science. One inexpensive but imprecise approach is to study established services in other areas. The greater the similarities between the communities or countries being compared, the more likely it is that the demand rates and trends in the new service will be similar, assuming that the services will be similarly organized. Information on waiting lists for existing services and rates of abortion among high-parity women can enhance and reinforce these estimates.

A more precise but more expensive approach to forecasting demand for sterilization uses household surveys and registers. This technique is employed in some primary health care services, particularly those with community-based outreach components involving routine, periodic household visits by trained community workers. All households or a systematic sample of households in the catchment area are visited to collect information about several critical variables that describe the health profile of each household. For family planning services, information is usually collected on family size, sex of children, age of youngest child, past and present contraceptive practice, and childbearing intentions (desire for additional children and the current number of children in relation to the "ideal" family size as stated by each respondent). Such information can be maintained in registers by community workers and updated periodically through further visits.

Analysis of consolidated household survey data can yield considerable information on the number of couples who may be likely clients of sterilization services. The household survey and register system allows community workers to be more efficient in meeting the specific contraceptive needs of each household, and subsequent surveys or reviews of field-worker registers may be used to evaluate the impact of family planning services.

A third approach to estimating potential case-load is presented in Table 9. This technique involves analysing data from censuses and surveys of contraceptive prevalence; it is convenient and cost-effective if recent data are available. However, even in an environment where sterilization is very well accepted, many eligible couples will not choose this procedure. Thus, estimates derived from this technique will need to be adjusted accordingly.

When services are first introduced into a community, requests for female sterilization may be limited. However, the case-load

Table 9. Estimating the potential case-load for sterilization[a]

	Value	Data source
	Formula: $n = a - (b + c + d)$	
$n =$	the number of couples who may want to choose vasectomy or female sterilization	
$a =$	the total number of couples of reproductive age who express a desire for no more children	Fertility or contraceptive prevalence surveys, plus census data
$b =$	the number of infertile couples	Fertility or contraceptive prevalence surveys
$c =$	the number of couples already protected by either female sterilization or vasectomy	Fertility or contraceptive prevalence surveys
$d =$	the number of couples who are ineligible because of service criteria (e.g., age and parity requirements)	Depends on service criteria (age and parity data may be obtained from the national census)

[a] This method yields an estimate of the number of couples who may want either vasectomy or female sterilization.

can be expected to increase as the number of satisfied clients grows, as accurate information becomes increasingly widespread, and as fears are allayed and misconceptions corrected. Having some idea of the potential number of clients can assist service managers in forecasting and planning for growth rather than being overcome by it.

Developing client-responsive services

All of the activities outlined in Table 8 are essential to the organization of female sterilization services. However, they may not be sufficient by themselves to ensure that services truly satisfy the needs of clients and are thus judged successful by the community. Public health professionals have considered the question of what makes for success in a particular service. The main features of successful family planning services have been identified as follows (Edmunds et al., 1987):

- Providing a wide choice of methods of contraception
- Placing the concept of family planning within the broader context of each client's experience
- Ensuring accessibility of family planning methods through a variety of staff and delivery systems
- Supporting clients by providing full information and counselling, and reassurance when problems arise
- Enhancing the quality of services by promoting the highest possible standards of care appropriate to the setting
- Responding to clients' needs and preferences for methods and services
- Providing effective outreach and follow-up
- Encouraging active client participation at all stages of service development and implementation
- Undertaking research and evaluation to elicit clients' perceptions and preferences

Satisfied clients are an important source of promotion and referrals for female sterilization services (see pages 49 and 54). If clients are treated with attentiveness and compassion by clinic staff, they will be more likely to leave with a favourable impression and to share that impression with potential clients, even if their surgery was difficult or complicated.

Female sterilization services should be located as close as possible to the community they are designed to serve. Some services have had good results by employing staff who reside in the community being served. Wherever possible, staff should have the same cultural and ethnic characteristics as their clients. The services should also have good connections with other local institutions, such as social welfare organizations, local health facilities, community-based family planning services, and local government councils or groups. In sum, sterilization services should strive to be fully integrated into the local community.

5. Financial management and budgeting

In order to provide services efficiently and to ensure their continuation, managers need to understand and use the principles of budgeting and other aspects of financial planning and management.

Determining costs and budgeting

In budgeting for sterilization services, it is important to distinguish nonrecurring and capital costs from recurring costs, and to budget for these separately. Table 10 lists typical cost categories for budget planning purposes.

Costs depend on local conditions and the characteristics of the service. For example, both the case-load and the surgical technique used will influence the budget requirements. Laparoscopy is more expensive than minilaparotomy, because of the costs of the special equipment needed, spare parts, and maintenance. On the other hand, these costs may be offset in a tertiary facility dealing with a large number of cases, because laparoscopy may require less of a surgeon's time. The provision of postpartum sterilization in a maternity setting is cost-effective because it generally requires less investment in space, personnel, and supplies than other means of service-delivery. In budget planning, managers should compare the costs of alternative approaches (e.g., paying surgeons per session or by salary, providing different types of information and education programmes) when deciding on the most cost-effective way to provide services.

It is possible to calculate the average cost of sterilization on a per case basis, taking into account both recurring and nonrecurring costs. Factors to consider include costs that are directly associated with serving clients, such as those for expendable supplies, clinical and surgical staff time spent in direct care, and equipment and other nonexpendable materials used. Other costs not directly associated with serving clients need to be

Table 10. Typical cost categories for budget planning for sterilization services

Capital and nonrecurring costs[a]

Space[b]
Equipment and nonexpendable supplies
Personnel training
Development of forms
Development and testing of information activities and materials
Surveys and special studies

Recurring costs

Space[b]
Personnel compensation and benefits
Pharmaceutical and expendable clinical supplies
Support services (e.g., cleaning, laundry, laboratory tests, bookkeeping, banking, audit)
Supervision, monitoring, and evaluation
Information and education activities
Refresher and in-service training activities
Reprinting of standard forms and information materials
Maintenance and taxes
Utilities (e.g., electricity, water)
Communications
Office supplies
Transport

[a] In calculating budgets and individual costs per client, capital costs are sometimes prorated over the anticipated life span of the investment.
[b] Space can represent either a capital cost (if purchased, constructed, or renovated) or a recurring cost (if leased).

included; these indirect, or "overhead", costs include salaries of administrative, managerial, and support staff, rent, utilities, and communications. The average cost per case is calculated by adding the costs for all of these factors for a given time period and dividing by the number of clients served during the same period. (Since resources such as staff and facilities are often used to provide a variety of family planning and health services, it is necessary to estimate the proportion of their total costs that can be attributed to the sterilization service.) Periodic calculation of the average cost per case allows the manager to monitor the costs and efficiency of the service. Furthermore, the costs of different means of service delivery (e.g., stationary versus mobile services, inpatient versus outpatient) and different sterilization techniques (e.g., minilaparotomy versus laparoscopy) can be assessed by refining and adapting these methods (McBride et al., 1987).

Financing services

Following the development of a budget, or alternative budgets, the next step is to finance the services. This is a relatively simple process if the service costs are included in the yearly allocation from the national treasury. Otherwise, financing services can be a complex problem involving multiple sources of funding. The latter situation is often faced by nongovernmental organizations and by private, for-profit service providers. The most common sources of funds for sterilization services are discussed below.

Government subsidies

Many national governments subsidize sterilization services as an integral part of their health and family planning services. Some governments (particularly in Asia) provide per-case subsidies, which may cover the full cost of sterilization. These payments may be made directly to institutions to defray the costs they incur in providing services, or they may go to individual providers. Some national health or family planning services compensate clients for costs incurred in undergoing sterilization, such as transportation and time lost from work. While subsidy schemes may enhance the availability and performance of sterilization services, they are often difficult to administer, may be susceptible to abuse or fraud (see pages 75 and 76), and could be difficult to sustain over the long term.

Grants from donor agencies

Several international donor agencies provide grants to governments, nongovernmental organizations, and other organizations involved with sterilization services. These grants are usually given to help establish and offer services during the first few years of operation. A list of these donor agencies is provided in Annex 1. Most have policies to phase out support and to encourage self-sufficiency and sustainability of services.

Client fees for service

Many health services are self-financing through fees paid by clients. Although the initial cost of sterilization is relatively high compared with temporary methods of contraception, the procedure is very cost-effective, since there are no recurring costs. Client fees must be set at a level which covers the costs, but not so high that they discourage use of the service. This may require an innovative approach to setting client fees, or to subsidizing services, in order not to deny services to clients. For example, some services have established "sliding-fee scales", in which the fees are set according to the clients' ability to pay, while others have allowed payments to be made by periodic instalments.

While no client should be denied services because of an inability to pay, it has been argued that all clients should be charged at least a nominal fee, since by contributing to the costs, the client gives an indication that the operation was chosen voluntarily.

Insurance schemes

Private insurance companies, health maintenance organizations, or government health insurance schemes may cover the cost of sterilization. These schemes generally recognize that sterilization costs are an investment in preventive health care, resulting in lower future costs from additional pregnancies or pregnancy-related health problems.

Income-generating schemes

Nongovernmental, not-for-profit organizations sometimes adopt income-generating schemes to help support the costs of sterilization. These organizations may undertake special fund-raising events, or they may subsidize the costs of sterilization using profit from temporary family planning or other reproductive health services.

Combined financing mechanisms

The most typical financing pattern for nongovernmental services is a combination of different sources. For example, PROFAMILIA, the nongovernmental national family planning organization of Colombia, relies on a combination of sliding-fee scales, profit from other family planning and health services, local fund-raising, and grants from donor agencies to pay for the costs of delivering sterilization services. This strategy allows PROFAMILIA to keep fees to clients low and affordable.

Financial management and audit

Services should also pay attention to financial management and accounting procedures. Effective accounting and auditing systems help managers to keep costs under control, to stay within budgets, and to avoid or anticipate financial difficulties. Governmental and other external donors often require particular accounting systems. In any case, all services should maintain internal accounting systems that are designed to permit periodic internal and external audit of the funds.

Planning for self-sufficiency

One important advantage of sterilization is its cost-effectiveness in relation to other methods of contraception (Huber & Harvey, 1989). Nevertheless, the costs of sterilization are immediate and relatively high, whereas those associated with most temporary methods are spread over a long period. In many countries and in poor communities with relatively little access to sizeable amounts of expendable income, most clients cannot afford the cost of sterilization, and costs for these clients must therefore be subsidized.

Because it is expensive to establish sterilization services and the costs are not usually covered by client fees, services may find their financial situation precarious, particularly during the first few years of operation. New services often rely on outside funding or on sources of income that may be unreliable for the long term, such as government subsidies or external donors. Therefore, managers must prepare for the future and continuously monitor and improve the efficiency, and thereby the sustainability, of services.

Different service-delivery sectors face somewhat different challenges in planning for sustainability. For many government health services, the goal is to disengage from multilateral and bilateral funding and to include the costs in annual government health budgets at the national or state level or in social security schemes. However, health budgets are often among the first to be reduced in times of economic hardship, and services should therefore seek to reduce costs and transfer remaining costs to other sources of income, such as client fees or private-sector insurance.

Nongovernmental, not-for-profit organizations usually depend on a variety of sources of income to support sterilization services, especially in the early years of operation. For such organizations, working towards self-sufficiency may be a more or less continuous process of compensating for reductions in one or another source of funding. Whenever possible, the long-term strategy should be to transfer the costs to clients or third parties. In any case, it is advisable for nongovernmental organizations to diversify and balance their sources of funding so that the elimination of any one source will not drastically affect overall fiscal health.

Finally, in most for-profit enterprises the sustainability mandate is clear: costs must be transferred to clients or recovered from third parties (such as insurance companies or governments) as soon as possible, or the institution will be forced to close. Governments and donors may be willing to support for-profit organizations during their early stages, especially with capital investment costs, but will not usually provide funds indefinitely for recurring costs.

Possible actions and strategies which may be considered by managers in working towards self-sufficiency are discussed briefly below.

Analysing and containing costs. Keeping costs to their absolute minimum without sacrificing quality is an obvious and prudent objective. The first step in deciding how to contain or reduce costs is to calculate the average cost per case and to determine the contributions of various factors that affect total costs (see page 40). Preparation of detailed annual budgets, review of expense reports, audits, and special cost studies are all useful managerial tools in analysing costs.

Reviewing service options. The way sterilization services are delivered and the techniques that are chosen have significant implications for costs and the sustainability of services. Some service options, grouped according to their relative costs, are listed in Table 11.

Achieving economies of scale. The average per-case cost of delivering sterilization services in a given setting generally falls

Table 11. Relative cost of various service options for female sterilization

Usually less expensive	*Usually more expensive*
Integrated, multipurpose services	Vertical, single-purpose services
Postpartum services	Interval services
Stationary service delivery	Mobile service delivery
Minilaparotomy	Laparoscopy
Tubal occlusion using ligation	Tubal occlusion using mechanical devices (clips, bands)
Local anaesthesia	General and regional anaesthesia
Outpatient services	Inpatient services
Nonexpendable supplies	Expendable supplies
Locally manufactured equipment and supplies	Imported equipment and supplies

as the number of clients increases. This is because the fixed costs are shared among more cases. Thus, a well-used service may be more sustainable.

Working towards cost recovery. Transferring costs by gradually increasing reliance on fee-for-service and insurance schemes is a prudent strategy for most sterilization services.

Adopting supplementary income-generating schemes. As mentioned earlier, many services subsidize the cost of sterilization by using profit from other family planning and health services and other income-generating schemes. Special fund-raising activities in the community may also be effective. One potential disadvantage of income-generating schemes is that they may distract managers from their primary task of providing high-quality health and family planning services.

6. Informing clients about female sterilization

Essential concepts

This chapter and the next discuss how women learn and make decisions about voluntary sterilization. The two chapters are intended to be read and used together.

Informing clients about female sterilization and other methods of contraception is different from promoting family planning or counselling clients. While each of these activities has its own primary purpose, individual staff members are often responsible for more than one of them. For instance, a nurse-midwife in a maternity service may inform and counsel clients. Likewise, a community worker may promote the practice of family planning and inform people about the various contraceptive methods. Whatever their individual responsibilities, staff members should understand the differences between these three activities.

Information	To provide facts about available methods of family planning
Promotion	To encourage people to practise family planning
Counselling	To assist the individual client to make an informed, voluntary, and well-considered decision about family planning

Information

The major purpose of information activities is to provide facts that the client can use in making a decision about family planning. Accordingly, clients must be given complete, accurate, and unbiased information about the available methods of contraception. Messages that favour one method of contraception over another, or that address only the advantages of particular methods, are misleading and compromise informed choice. In the case of female sterilization, the procedure's intended permanence must be stressed.

For information activities to be effective, a range of family planning services must be available and accessible to the public and provided in a non-coercive atmosphere. If a family planning service provides information about female sterilization but the procedure is either unavailable or inaccessible, potential clients will be disappointed and frustrated, and the credibility of the family planning service will be damaged. If information is presented in a coercive atmosphere, clients are likely not to believe it and to resist female sterilization, whereas they might have considered it in a more open and supportive environment. If clients undergoing sterilization feel pressured in any way, they are likely to regret the procedure afterwards and to criticize both the method and the provider.

Family planning providers must ensure that all personnel who provide information about contraception are themselves well informed. Facts about methods, their advantages and disadvantages, and their side-effects should be incorporated in training programmes for doctors, nurses, field-workers, counsellors, and other appropriate personnel. Staff members should also be routinely supervised to ensure that they are providing clients with accurate and complete information.

Promotion

The major purpose of promotion, or motivation, is to encourage people to practise family planning. It is acceptable to promote the benefits of small families and to encourage clients to use some method of family planning. However, urging healthy clients to use specific methods compromises voluntary choice (WFHAAVSC, 1987).

Family planning services have undertaken a variety of promotional activities. One of the most common is to use trained community workers to promote contraception; these individuals usually have other public health or family planning responsibilities, such as providing information about health services and methods of contraception, distributing contraceptive or medical supplies, or accompanying clients to clinics.

Some promotional activities, notably provision of incentives and disincentives, can pose serious threats to free and informed choice (see page 75).

Counselling

The purpose of counselling is to assist the client to make an informed, voluntary, well-considered decision regarding family planning. In addition to providing information about methods of contraception (filling in gaps in the client's knowledge and correcting misconceptions), the counsellor focuses on the client's decision and how it is made (see Chapter 7 for further details). When discussing sterilization, the counsellor must stress that the method is intended to be permanent.

Developing information activities and materials for clients

Information activities and materials about female sterilization for clients require careful planning and implementation. In particular, the audience must be defined carefully in order to permit the development of appropriate messages, the identification of the most appropriate channels for conveying them, and the evaluation of the effectiveness of the activities.

Informed and voluntary choice is jeopardized when undue emphasis is placed on particular methods of contraception. Information about sterilization should be part of a broad communication programme about family planning, and clients should therefore receive information about all the available options before they make a choice.

As providers plan and develop information activities and materials, they should seek assistance from two valuable sources: members of the target audience and professionals with experience in communication activities. Client participation is essential if the programme is to succeed. Through focus groups and interviews, clients can help develop the messages to be conveyed, and identify the appropriate information channels for these messages. Furthermore, they can review sketches and drafts of materials being developed during the critical pretesting stage.

A variety of professionals have considerable experience with information activities and should be asked to participate in planning and carrying out the programme. Managers should draw upon the experience of personnel from areas such as health education, communications, graphic design, advertising, production of audiovisual materials, and communications research. Their efforts can encourage better use of resources and can enhance the effectiveness of information materials and activities.

Family planning managers who are inexperienced in carrying out information programmes, and those in countries where resources are scarce, may have difficulty in obtaining appropriate professional assistance. Ministries of health, major hospitals, and family planning organizations often have communication departments that can help to plan and develop information programmes. In addition, several specialized organizations (such as the Program for Appropriate Technology in Health, and Population Communication Services) have provided training and technical assistance to family planning services in developing countries. The addresses of these agencies are listed in Annex 1.

The major steps in developing information activities and materials are described in the box opposite. Careful analysis of the community is the first step in any successful information programme (see pages 35 and 47). During this stage, staff should talk to clients and should examine the messages that are being circulated about female sterilization. Clients receive information about contraception (including female sterilization) in many ways. Some of that information may be inaccurate or incomplete.

Service managers should also examine the context in which they are communicating. They should seek to answer the following questions:

- What rumours and myths exist?
- What forces are at work that might make clients resist or disbelieve information about family planning, including female sterilization?
- Which sources of information does the community trust and rely upon?
- What information is being presented in newspapers, on television, and on radio?
- Is family planning widely practised in the community, or is it just beginning to be used?
- How prevalent is female sterilization?
- Are there any laws or local customs that might restrict public discussion about family planning and female sterilization?

Major steps in developing an information programme about female sterilization[a]

1. *Analysis*

   Research the proposed target audiences and their characteristics. Determine what messages are circulating and what materials already exist. Examine the institution's ability to carry out the information programme, and consider if additional resources are required.

2. *Developing a plan*

   Determine the objectives, topics, and target audiences. Identify the resources required, both inside and outside the institution. Identify staff members who will be involved, and spell out their responsibilities. Develop a schedule and a budget.

3. *Developing messages*

   Investigate the target audiences' knowledge about family planning. Develop messages based on these results. Review these messages with staff.

4. *Developing materials and activities*

   Select the most appropriate information channels to convey the messages. Design materials and activities, and review these with staff.

5. *Pretesting and revising*

   Pretest the messages, materials, and activities on the target audiences. Revise as necessary and review the revised materials and activities with staff. Repeat this stage as required.

6. *Implementation*

   Train staff members to use the materials and to carry out the activities. Produce and distribute the materials. Implement the programme.

7. *Evaluation*

   Assess the impact of the information activities on the target audiences. Revise the material and activities as required.

[a] Sources: Population Communication Services & Population Information Program, and Program for Appropriate Technology in Health, 1988.

- What is the role of women in the society, and how does it affect information activities about family planning?
- What role do men play in making decisions about family planning?
- Are other agencies already providing information about contraception and female sterilization?

To obtain answers to these questions, service providers can interview community leaders and clients, talk to experienced health personnel who have worked in the community, consult reference materials, and conduct surveys and focus groups. A major goal of all these activities is to collect information about the proposed target audiences so that messages can be tailored to meet their needs.

During the analysis stage, the institution's ability to carry out the proposed information programme should also be examined. Staff should evaluate whether outside assistance is needed.

After careful analysis of the community and service context, the second step is to develop a plan. This stage is concerned with identifying the objectives and topics of the programme. Staff members select the segments of the client population that will be the target of the information programme, and then obtain additional information about those groups. The following questions should be considered:

- Are these potential clients literate, partially literate, or illiterate?
- What languages do they speak and read?
- What do they already know about family planning and female sterilization?
- What concerns, questions, and misconceptions do they have about family planning and female sterilization?
- Who influences their decisions about family planning?
- What is the desired family size?
- What is important to the audience?
- What problems are they facing?

Again, interviews, surveys, focus groups, and reference materials can help provide answers to these questions. Staff members responsible for information activities should describe the target audience in writing, revise that description as the activities progress, and continually refer to it as a guide. For example: "The primary target audience is rural, illiterate, married women aged over 30 and under 45 with at least two children. Secondary target audiences are their husbands and in-laws."

At step 2, staff should also determine what resources are needed to carry out the information programme. Such resources include skills in advertising, marketing, graphics, writing, production of audiovisual materials, and printing. Service managers should identify which staff will be involved in developing and implementing the information programme, and produce the schedules and budgets needed to manage the activities.

Once the target audience has been selected and its characteristics, needs, attitudes, and level of understanding assessed, key messages should be developed (step 3). These should address the main topics identified during audience research. When the messages have been determined, staff should select the most appropriate information channels (see page 54) to convey these messages and begin designing materials and activities (step 4).

The next step is to pretest the materials and activities with the target audience (step 5). Pretesting is essential, since it helps to ensure that information materials and activities are culturally appropriate, relevant to clients' concerns, and presented in familiar language and at an educational level that clients can understand.

Pretesting can be conducted in a variety of ways. Under the guidance of a trained leader, focus groups of 8–10 people can provide feedback about messages and illustrations, and the clarity of concepts and language. Alternatively, staff can conduct structured, in-depth interviews with individuals; this technique enables individuals to respond without being influenced by others' opinions. One convenient way of pretesting is to interview members of the target audience at a common gathering place, such as a clinic waiting room.

Managers should plan for several rounds of pretesting when developing an information programme. The process can take from a few days to several months, depending upon the skills of staff and outside experts, the complexity of the information materials and activities, and the number of changes needed. Insisting that pretesting be rushed will be detrimental to the information programme. Elements that require pretesting include illustrations, text, layout, size, colour, and sequence (for printed materials) and script, recorded voices, music, and images (for slide programmes, videos, and films) (Zimmerman & Perkin, 1982).

While they cannot provide the client's perspective, health care professionals have an important role to play as messages are developed and pretested: they can comment on the accuracy and completeness of material, and their guidance is essential when medical or scientific information is being prepared. At the same time, the results of audience pretesting can help these staff learn how to improve the ways in which they communicate with clients.

Once pretest results have been collected, the messages, materials, and activities are revised as needed. If revisions are extensive, another round of pretesting may be required.

Implementation may begin as soon as the information activities and materials have been revised and finalized (step 6). This phase involves such tasks as training staff, producing an adequate supply of materials for service sites, establishing an efficient reordering system, scheduling broadcasts and events in a cost-effective way and at times that are most convenient for the target audience, and providing audiovisual equipment and training to service sites. All activities should be monitored and supervised throughout this stage to ensure that the objectives are being achieved and the target audiences are being reached.

The final step is to review the programme and to use that assessment to decide on future activities (step 7). Information programmes are cyclical in nature, and the steps presented above should be repeated in response to the changing needs of the audiences and the environment.

Information channels

Clients acquire information by hearing or seeing it expressed in different ways at different times. They listen to friends, neighbours, health care workers, and community leaders. If they are literate, they may read pamphlets, magazines, and newspapers. If they are partially literate or illiterate, they may ask other people to read material to them. They may also watch television or listen to the radio, see poster and billboard displays, or attend information sessions at health care centres and in their communities. Because people obtain information from so many different sources and because they learn by hearing and reading messages over and over again, it is generally more effective to use a combination of information channels than to rely on only one (Ross et al., 1989).

Before choosing the channels to be used, it is essential to define the target audience and identify the objectives and messages of the information programme (see page 49). A particular channel should be selected because it is an effective and efficient way to reach the audience and accomplish the programme's goals. Planners should also consider how to evaluate the effectiveness and costs of particular information channels.

Several channels that have been used to convey information to clients about female sterilization are described in the box overleaf. Some of these channels rely on interpersonal communication, i.e., individuals talking to other individuals or to small groups of people. Some rely on technology, such as printing or electronic media. The most important channel is the communication that occurs between the client and the provider. Accordingly, the provider should always speak directly to the client, even if other channels are used.

All of the information channels described overleaf have costs associated with them—for instance, salaries or time away from other tasks for staff involved; fees for outside experts; and costs for paper, ink, photography, videotape, or air time. The costs of using a particular channel must be weighed against its effectiveness in disseminating information to potential clients.

Clinic-based information activities

Outpatient services, antenatal clinics, postpartum clinics, primary health care facilities, and family planning clinics often provide a range of information to clients about health-related subjects, including female sterilization. Information sessions, sometimes with audiovisual presentations, should be conducted in private rooms or in quiet waiting areas. Brochures may be displayed and distributed, and posters hung on the walls. Service providers must ensure that staff responsible for these activities are fully knowledgeable and well trained, that clients have an opportunity to ask questions, and that the atmosphere is conducive to individual decision-making.

Antenatal clinics are particularly appropriate sites for providing information about nutrition, immunization, and family planning, including female sterilization. A pregnant woman may be thinking about which method of contraception to use after giving

Information channels that can be used to inform people about female sterilization

Interpersonal communication between the provider and client
Enables the provider to establish a personal relationship with the client and to ensure that she is well informed.
Disadvantages: may be time-consuming. Providers may lack appropriate training and may underestimate the need for interpersonal communication. Clients may be reluctant to ask questions and to make decisions independently.

Community-based field-workers[a]
Often trusted and respected sources of information. Can provide information about a range of health services, including family planning. May also refer clients to services and provide follow-up.
Disadvantages: must be closely supervised to ensure that they do not pressure clients and that they provide accurate, complete information.

Satisfied clients
Often trusted and respected sources of information because of their close links with the community. Particularly valuable when female sterilization is being introduced, when the community is resistant to it, or when public discussion of tubal occlusion is considered unacceptable.
Disadvantages: must be closely supervised to ensure that they do not pressure potential clients and that they provide accurate, complete information.

Printed materials
Can be used to answer common questions and concerns and to serve as reference materials. May be designed to support presentations by health workers (e.g., flip charts) or to be used independently (e.g., brochures, posters).
Disadvantages: must present information in a straightforward, non-technical manner without condescending to clients; should be visually appealing and tailored to literacy levels and needs of the target audience. May be expensive to produce.

Traditional media
Use accepted traditions (e.g., folk drama, songs, dances and puppetry) to communicate health messages. Messages can be developed and delivered by local groups, which can help to overcome resistance to new ideas. Useful in rural areas.
Disadvantages: if content and quality of performances vary, may not convey the chosen messages effectively.

Audiovisual materials
Examples include films, filmstrips, videotapes, audiotapes, slides and overhead transparencies. Can be especially interesting and appealing

to clients when they combine words, music and colourful images. May be shown in waiting rooms.
Disadvantages: must present information in a straightforward, non-technical manner without condescending to clients. May be costly to purchase or produce (if produced outside the community may not meet the needs of the target audience, if produced locally require personnel with advanced knowledge of communications and technology). Need reliable sources of electricity, special equipment and trained personnel.

Mass media
Examples include newspapers, magazines, radio, television, billboards, posters, and advertisements. Can be used to inform the general public about female sterilization. Most useful channel for reaching a large target audience.
Disadvantages: May be inappropriate if sterilization is considered an unacceptable topic for public discussion. Can be costly to produce (if produced locally require personnel with advanced knowledge of communications and technology). May provide only limited coverage in rural areas. Messages are usually simple.

Professional networks
Can help to educate professionals about female sterilization, serve as sources of referral, and can sometimes provide sterilization services to clients. Such networks include doctors, registered midwives, nurses, teachers, social workers, religious leaders, and other community service professionals who come into contact with the target audience. May be reached through seminars, letters, presentations, and announcements in professional journals and newsletters.
Disadvantages: require regular, close contact with the target audience to be effective.

Community groups and organizations
Community groups and organizations in which women predominate can help to inform women in the community about female sterilization, and can also serve as sources of referral. Examples include mothers' clubs, cooperatives, women's agricultural organizations, professional organizations, and social clubs. These groups may be reached through satisfied clients, presentations at group meetings, or handouts. Men's organizations may also be used in settings where female sterilization is being introduced, where opposition is strong, or where women have limited authority to make decisions.
Disadvantages: require regular, close contact with the target audience to be effective.

[a] See Table 12 for guidelines about using community-based field-workers.

Table 12. Guidelines for using community-based field-workers

Activity
1. Train field-workers so that they are fully knowledgeable about all available methods of contraception.
2. Ensure that field-workers understand their role: providing information and assistance to help clients make their own independent choices.
3. Teach field-workers to be unbiased when they present information about different methods of contraception.
4. Train field-workers to discuss *all* available methods with clients.
5. Train field-workers to answer routine questions that clients may have.
6. Teach field-workers to respect the private nature of decisions about contraception.
7. Train field-workers to know when to refer clients for further information.
8. Supervise field-workers carefully and retrain them as needed.
Field-workers should not
1. Be paid according to the number of clients they refer for sterilization.
2. Be required to meet targets for sterilization referrals.
3. Have their job performance evaluated according to the number of clients who choose sterilization.
4. Conduct aggressive promotional activities that focus on sterilization.

birth. If she is considering sterilization, the antenatal period gives her time to think carefully about the decision and to discuss it with her spouse. It also allows the woman and the facility to plan for the surgery if it is to be performed postpartum. At the same time, special precautions must be taken if a client chooses tubal occlusion during pregnancy, since her ability to make a carefully considered decision may be compromised by physical or emotional factors (see page 61).

Counteracting misinformation

Misinformation about family planning methods is a major obstacle to contraceptive use in some countries (Gallen et al., 1987). The effects of different methods of contraception are often the subject of rumours and myths (e.g., "female sterilization makes a woman stop menstruating"). Sometimes misinformation may be circulated by dissatisfied clients, opponents of family planning services, or even poorly informed health providers.

Broad-based information activities that communicate in a simple, clear, and objective manner can be used to counteract rumours and myths about female sterilization and other methods of contraception. Service providers should aim to identify any such rumours and misinformation as soon as possible and address them at the source; follow up clients who are using methods of contraception to ensure that they possess correct information; provide services of high quality that are trusted by the community; provide accurate information about contraceptives, including their advantages and disadvantages; and use words and symbols in information activities that promote understanding, rather than confusion (Rogers, 1973).

7. The individual decision about female sterilization[1]

This chapter focuses on the individual woman's decision about female sterilization. Because the factors bearing on this decision vary from client to client, service providers must be prepared to help each woman as she makes her choice according to her particular needs. The provider should take every possible measure to ensure that the decision for or against sterilization is made thoughtfully and voluntarily, on the basis of complete information about the procedure, including its risks, benefits, and alternatives.

Personal decision-making

Individual decisions about fertility and contraception are made for a variety of reasons. They are influenced by personal circumstances, such as family size, economic situation, and health status. They are also affected by the context in which the person lives (for instance, cultural expectations about family formation and size, public policies, and information and education available about family planning).

As the circumstances of their lives change, people make different contraceptive choices. Some couples begin by using temporary methods, such as the pill or condoms, to space pregnancies. As the years pass, these couples may switch from one method to another. They stop practising contraception altogether when they decide to have a child. Then, when they have had all the children they want, they may start thinking about long-lasting temporary methods (intrauterine devices, injectables, implantables) or methods intended to be permanent (tubal occlusion, vasectomy).

[1] Much of this chapter has been adapted from *Family planning counseling and voluntary sterilization: a guide for managers*, by G. S. Neamatalla & P. B. Harper, published by the Association for Voluntary Surgical Contraception, 1990.

Other couples only begin to think about using contraception when they have all the children they want. For these couples, voluntary sterilization is often an obvious and sensible choice; for some, it is the only method of contraception they will ever use.

The role of the service provider

Because tubal occlusion is intended to be permanent and involves surgery, with its associated risks, service providers must ensure that potential clients are given all the necessary information about the procedure and must help them to reach an independent decision.

The provider is responsible both for conducting general information activities (as described in Chapter 6), and for providing assistance to individual women who either are considering female sterilization or have decided to undergo the procedure. The focus of this chapter is on the second aspect—the individual woman.

Counselling should be offered to all women who express an interest in contraception. If a woman chooses sterilization after individual counselling, the provider needs to document her informed consent, prepare her for the operation, and give her instructions on how to prepare for surgery and what to expect during and after the operation. The goal of all these activities is to help ensure that the woman fully understands the method she has chosen and makes her decision voluntarily. Achieving this goal increases the likelihood that the woman will be satisfied with the choice she has made.

Family planning counselling

The purpose of family planning counselling is to help the client to make an informed, voluntary, and well-considered decision regarding fertility and contraception. The counsellor ensures that the client is informed about all available methods of contraception and helps her apply this knowledge to her circumstances. Fig. 4 illustrates how family planning counselling fits into the client's decision-making process. Counselling is particularly important for sterilization because the method involves surgery and is intended to be permanent. It is a critical checkpoint between the client's decision to seek sterilization and

Fig. 4. Client decision process concerning fertility

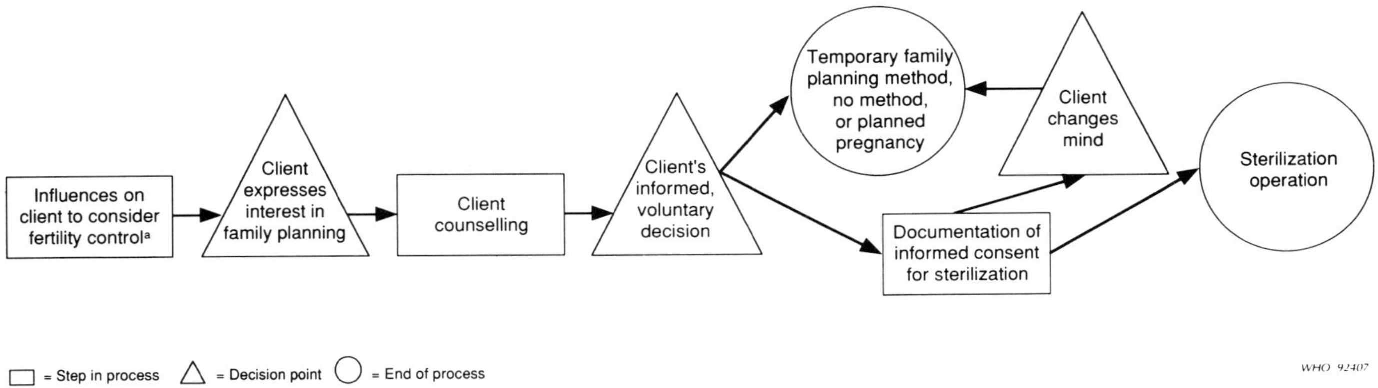

[a] Such influences may include information and education programmes, socioeconomic conditions, or peer pressure.

Adapted from Butta, 1988. Used by permission.

the succeeding steps that lead to surgery. With counselling, a wrong decision, made because a client is misinformed or under stress, can be averted or reversed.

While some components of counselling (such as the provision of information) can be conducted in group settings, every client must have an opportunity to raise questions and discuss her decision in private with a counsellor. Counselling involves two-way communication, with both the counsellor and the client spending time listening and talking. The counsellor should be objective, showing no bias for or against female sterilization or any other family planning method. Whenever it is possible, the client's partner should also receive counselling. However, the partner's consent should not be a prerequisite for receiving services unless it is a legal requirement (see page 73).

Sometimes a client's choice may conflict with the wishes and interests of her spouse, her family, or even her community. In such circumstances, the service provider must ensure that the client fully understands how the people around her may react to her decision.

One of the principal aims of counselling is to identify clients who are likely to change their mind about sterilization after the procedure has been performed (see page 74). Several factors have been associated with dissatisfaction or other negative reactions after female sterilization, and should be discussed with the client before surgery (see overleaf). These factors should not be used as arbitrary grounds for denying sterilization to a client. However, clients who exhibit any of these characteristics require the most careful counselling (see page 74).

A client may also feel dissatisfied if she chooses tubal occlusion but is then unable to undergo the procedure. The counsellor should be aware of potential obstacles, such as unavailability of services, the client's inability to pay for the surgery, strict age and parity requirements, or a long waiting period.

Who provides counselling?

Family planning counselling may be provided by doctors, nurses, paramedical staff, other health workers, or any other person who has received appropriate training. While counsellors require special training, they do not have to be professional psychologists, therapists, or social workers. They should, however, be able to recognize signs of any serious psychological problem and know how to refer clients as necessary.

Client characteristics associated with dissatisfaction and other negative reactions following female sterilization

- Being young[a]
- Having no or few[a] children
- Having children all of the same sex
- Having a child in poor health, especially the youngest
- Being in an unstable marriage or having an uncooperative spouse
- Being single or widowed
- Being pressured by the spouse or someone else to have a sterilization
- Making the decision when under unusual stress (e.g., during labour or shortly after the death of a child)
- Making the decision quickly, without time to reflect and reconsider
- Lacking access to other methods of contraception
- Having unresolved religious or other cultural conflicts
- Receiving payments or other incentives that may unduly influence the decision (see page 75)
- Being incompletely or incorrectly informed about female sterilization
- Having health reasons for ending childbearing (see page 72)
- Having unfulfilled maternal desires
- Having unrealistic expectations about sterilization and its consequences
- Relying on the possibility of reversal as a factor in the decision for sterilization
- Having unresolved feelings about wanting more children in the event of remarriage or the death of a child

[a] Definition may vary, depending upon a variety of cultural and social factors.

Effective counselling requires good observational, speaking, and listening skills. Counsellors should be fully informed about all methods of contraception and able to communicate that information in a language and in terms that clients can understand.

Regardless of who counsels the client, the operating surgeon must use professional judgement to ensure that the woman has made an informed, voluntary, well-considered decision. The surgeon may speak directly to the client before she is sedated or may verify that counselling has been given by speaking to the staff responsible and checking the client record, including the informed-consent form (Neamatalla & Harper, 1990).

Sometimes health personnel receive payments or benefits when they refer clients for voluntary sterilization or perform the surgery; at other times job performance is judged on the basis of the number of family planning clients staff recruit or the number of sterilization procedures they perform. Such individuals are not appropriate counsellors, because they have a personal interest in the client's decision and may be inclined to encourage the woman to choose tubal occlusion.

In some countries, method-specific promoters work in the community, providing information about individual methods of contraception. They should not counsel family planning clients, since their narrow focus is in conflict with the counsellor's responsibility to help the client choose from among a variety of contraceptive options.

How is counselling given?

The following activities should be part of every family planning counselling session:

- Welcome the client in a friendly and helpful manner.
- Ask the client to specify her family planning goals.
- Determine what the client already knows about contraception.
- Provide information about contraceptive methods and services as required.
- Determine the client's circumstances and the factors influencing her choice of contraception.
- Encourage the client to ask questions and discuss her concerns.
- Correct any misconceptions regarding methods of contraception.

- Help the client make an informed, voluntary, and well-considered decision.
- Provide more detailed information if the client selects a method (in the case of sterilization, this would include instructions on how to prepare for surgery, and what to expect during and after the operation, as detailed on page 71 and in Annex 2).
- Arrange appointments and provide for follow-up as needed.

Counsellors usually rely on illustrations, brochures, posters, flip charts, anatomical models, or examples of contraceptives to help them explain the various contraceptive options. If clients are at risk of HIV infection, the counsellor should also provide information about the prevention of AIDS.

The duration and depth of counselling sessions vary, depending upon how much each client already knows and how certain she is about her choice. If a client interested in sterilization arrives at the counselling session with all the relevant information and has had time to consider the decision carefully, counselling may be relatively brief. On the other hand, if she has only recently learned about female sterilization or has made the decision for surgery quickly, counselling may take longer because the counsellor will need to provide more information and discuss the decision more extensively.

When accurate information about sterilization and other methods of contraception is widely available, it is likely that clients will come to the service site relatively well informed and ready to make a decision. Extensive counselling may be required in the following situations:

- when sterilization services are new,
- when the general public knows little about tubal occlusion and other methods of contraception,
- when information circulating in the community is poor,
- when providers emphasize a particular method of contraception.

The counsellor should listen to the client carefully and encourage her to speak and ask questions throughout the counselling session. Counselling about female sterilization should cover the issues listed opposite.

1. Determine if the client meets eligibility criteria (see page 73).
2. Ensure that the client understands that sterilization involves surgery and is intended to be permanent.
3. Inform the client about other available methods of contraception, for both men and women. Tailor this information to the client's needs, depending upon what she already knows and what her family planning goals are.
4. Assess the client's decision and feelings about sterilization to determine if her choice is voluntary and well considered. Discuss possible life changes that might lead the client to change her mind about the procedure later (such as remarriage, loss of a child, or a change in economic status). Prepare the client for ending fertility.
5. If reversal services are well established in the service area, their existence is widely known, or the client raises the issue, inform her about the prospects for reversal (see Chapter 14). If the possibility of reversal is a factor in the client's decision for tubal occlusion, sterilization may be inappropriate.
6. If the client's decision appears to be involuntary or poorly considered, tell her that she seems likely to change her mind about sterilization after the procedure has been performed. Ask the client to spend more time thinking about the decision. Encourage her to use temporary methods of contraception in the meantime.
7. If the client's decision for sterilization appears to be informed, voluntary, and well considered, continue the counselling session.
    - Describe in detail the benefits, risks, and side-effects of sterilization. Explain that tubal occlusion has no effect on general health or sexual relations. Discuss the inherent risks of any surgical procedure (infection, bleeding, anaesthesia-related complications), as well as the risks specifically related to tubal occlusion, including the small possibility of complications, failure, and ectopic pregnancy.
    - Describe the surgical procedure and how it works. Explain what will happen in the operating theatre, and describe the likely post-operative effects. Tell the client how to prepare for surgery.
    - If appropriate, explain that sterilization does not provide protection against HIV infection.
    - Tell the client about any fees she is expected to pay.
    - Advise the client to use temporary contraception until surgery.
    - Tell the client that she is free to decide against sterilization at any time before the surgery is performed.
    - Complete informed-consent procedures.
    - Schedule appointments for medical screening and surgery, as needed.

Making the decision

The client may be counselled at any time once she decides to seek information about female sterilization. However, she should not choose to undergo tubal occlusion when physical or emotional factors may compromise her ability to make a carefully considered and informed decision. For example, a client should not choose sterilization when she is in labour, is sedated, or is experiencing stress before, during, or after a pregnancy-related event or procedure (Butta, 1988).

One consideration for a woman undergoing postpartum sterilization is the viability of the newborn. If a woman is counselled and makes the decision for sterilization during the antenatal period, the counsellor should determine whether she will still want to have a tubal occlusion if the baby is not healthy. The counsellor should record the woman's response. It is especially important to know the client's wishes if sterilization is scheduled to be performed at the same time as caesarean section.

If the newborn is unhealthy and the staff believe that the child's death might cause the woman to change her mind about sterilization, the procedure should be delayed for a minimum of 6 weeks (42 days). By that time, the health status of the baby will be clearer and the woman's uterus will have returned to its normal size. If she still wishes to have a sterilization, she can then undergo an interval procedure (see page 102). On the other hand, if the woman already has all the children she wants, she may definitely want to go ahead with the procedure, even if the newborn is unhealthy.

While it is important for the client to have sufficient time to reflect on the decision before surgery, arbitrary waiting periods are inadvisable, unless required by law. If the client was well informed before coming to the service site, she has usually had sufficient time to reflect on the decision; in such cases, it is unnecessary to impose another waiting period.

In some settings, especially when sterilization services are not conveniently located for clients, a mandatory waiting period often denies services to those who are unable to make two trips to the facility and is therefore discriminatory.

Waiting periods should be required only for clients who are not well informed when they come to the service site and who can return to the site without difficulty, and for clients who seem likely to change their mind about the decision after sterilization has been performed (Butta, 1988).

Family planning counselling and informed-consent procedures may take place days or even weeks before surgery. If considerable time elapses, however, staff members at the surgical facility should verify that the woman still wants to go ahead with the procedure and that she fully understands the nature of her decision.

Informed consent[1]

A client who has chosen tubal occlusion must give her informed consent. This means that she voluntarily authorizes the provider to perform the surgical procedure, and that she makes this authorization in full possession and understanding of the relevant facts.

In many countries, consent is documented in written form and signed by the client, the surgeon (or a representative of the surgeon), and a witness (this is particularly important if the client is not literate). Documentation of informed consent is often part of counselling. In many settings the consent form is considered the legal authorization to perform the surgery. However, consent procedures should not be regarded merely as a legal requirement or as a protective measure for the provider; they are an important means of protecting the client's right to make a voluntary, informed decision.

Some sterilization services use standard surgical consent forms developed for all types of surgery. Others use specially designed forms to ensure that the most important points related to female sterilization are included. Forms designed for female sterilization services should contain a statement that the client understands that sterilization is intended to be a permanent procedure, and if successful, will prevent any further pregnancies; that sterilization involves surgery, with its associated risks (including a slight chance of failure); that temporary methods of contraception are available; and that she may change her mind at any time before surgery (i.e., before the fallopian tubes are occluded), without any loss of medical or financial benefits.

A sample consent form is given in Fig. 5. However, each service will need to develop a form appropriate to the specific

---

[1] For more information about informed consent, see *Informed consent and voluntary sterilization,* by P. Butta, published by the Association for Voluntary Surgical Contraception, 1988.

Fig. 5. Sample informed-consent form for sterilization

I, ______________________, the undersigned, request that a steri-
client's name

lization via ______________________ be performed on my person.
specify the procedure

I make this request of my own free will, without having been forced or given any special inducement. I understand that:

1. Temporary methods of contraception are available to me and my partner.
2. The procedure involves surgery (the details of which have been explained to me).
3. This surgical procedure involves risks and benefits, both of which have been explained to me.
4. If the procedure is successful, I will be unable to have any more children.
5. The effect of the procedure is intended to be permanent.
6. I can decide against the procedure at any time before the operation is performed (and no medical, health, or other benefits or services will be withheld from me as a result).

______________________ ____________

Signature or mark of client — Date

______________________ ____________

Signature of attending physician or delegated assistant — Date

If the client cannot read, a witness chosen by the client, of the same sex and speaking the same language, must sign the following declaration:

I, the undersigned, attest to the fact that the client has affixed her thumbprint or mark in my presence.

______________________ ____________

Signature or mark of witness — Date

Adapted from Butta, 1988. Used by permission.

customs, regulations and laws in force locally. The form should be presented in a language and using terms that clients can understand. Pretesting is therefore required, as described on page 53.

If the client is either illiterate or only partially literate, a trained staff member should explain the details of the form to her and ensure that she fully understands the elements of informed consent. A trained interpreter should carry out this function if the form is not available in the client's own language. In order to avoid coercion and to ensure objective translation, interpreters should not be paid referral agents or people who accompany clients to the facility.

However, the presence of a client's signature or mark on an informed-consent form does not necessarily mean that she has requested the operation willingly or in full knowledge of the facts and options available. She may feel intimidated by friends, family members, or family planning providers, or be reluctant to express her concerns or raise questions. Particularly in societies where women traditionally exercise little decision-making authority, clients may be inclined to go along with the decision, rather than to resist or ask for more information. Providers must always be alert to signs that the woman is consenting to sterilization either against her wishes or without full information.

Preoperative and postoperative instructions

Instructions on how to prepare for surgery and what to expect during and after the operation are usually given during the counselling session or at the time of the preoperative examination. The staff member who provides this information must be familiar with the medical and surgical details associated with female sterilization.

Service staff should explain the surgical procedure and the anaesthesia to be used in simple, nontechnical terms. Because surgery can be an unfamiliar and frightening prospect, the woman should know that the procedure will be performed in an operating theatre by professional staff who will be wearing masks and operating gowns. If the woman will be awake during surgery, staff should tell her what pain or discomfort she may feel and how she can cooperate with the surgical team.

Clients also need to know what to do after surgery and how they can expect to feel in the days following the operation (see page 108). They must be told how to recognize signs of complications and what action to take if they occur. Postoperative information should be presented briefly before sedation and surgery, and reviewed in detail after surgery when the woman is fully awake and alert.

If a client lives some distance from the service site or if the surgery is performed in a mobile setting, it is especially important that she fully understands the postoperative instructions. In particular, she needs to know where to go if she has signs of complications.

Many sterilization providers have found it helpful to give simple written information to clients. This helps clients remember what they should do before and after surgery, and serves as a quick reference when they are at home. Written information can assist even partially literate or illiterate clients, since they often know people who can read the information to them. Annex 2 provides a sample of the type of information provided to clients who are planning to undergo sterilization. This material may or may not be illustrated. Additional copies should be available after surgery, in case the client has misplaced the material.

Ending childbearing for health reasons

For some clients, pregnancy poses a serious health risk (see page 78), and contraception is therefore recommended for medical reasons. Sterilization is often considered in these situations. As in other cases, these women should make voluntary, informed, well-considered decisions about contraception; family planning counselling is necessary. However, the nature of counselling is different when contraception has been recommended for medical reasons.

When a woman is advised to undergo sterilization for medical reasons, the doctor and other staff members must ensure that she understands the comparative risks associated with pregnancy, sterilization, and other methods of contraception. Vasectomy for the partner and long-term methods (intrauterine devices and implantable contraceptives) should also be considered, particularly if the sterilization surgery poses significant risks for the woman. If the woman chooses to undergo tubal occlusion, informed consent is necessary.

In a few instances sterilization is performed without family planning counselling and consent. For example, if a woman arrives at the hospital in shock due to a ruptured uterus, she must undergo emergency surgery, and a sterilization is often medically necessary because of the high risk of death if the woman becomes pregnant again. In such cases, postoperative counselling is essential to help the patient adjust to her loss of fertility and understand why the surgery was necessary.

Women who undergo sterilization for health reasons are likely to experience regret, dissatisfaction, and other negative reactions, particularly if they are not convinced that pregnancy would be dangerous for them. Some of them may want more children and be deeply saddened by the prospect of ending childbearing. Staff members should be sensitive to such feelings and should help these patients come to terms with the need to avoid pregnancy.

Denying services

Sterilization services may be denied to clients for three reasons.

1. The person has a medical condition that is a contraindication to surgery (see page 79). Such contraindications are usually temporary, and the procedure can be performed as soon as they are resolved. In some cases, the contraindication may make it necessary to refer the client to a better-equipped medical facility or to perform the procedure under general anaesthesia. Family planning counsellors should inform clients who are denied services because of temporary medical contraindications that they will be able to choose female sterilization at a later date if they wish to do so, and should advise them of the option to use temporary contraception in the meantime.

2. The client fails to meet the criteria, established through laws or regulations, related to age, parity, marital status or spousal consent (see page 8). Sometimes the surgeon has the authority to waive such restrictions. Family planning counsellors should be fully informed about such criteria and the procedures to follow regarding them; they may need to consult with other staff members before denying services. If the criteria are not mandatory, providers should avoid enforcing them arbitrarily and should apply them on the basis of the needs of the individual client. In particular, spousal consent should not be a prerequisite for services unless it is a legal requirement.

3. Staff believe the client is very likely to change her mind about sterilization or to have a negative reaction after the surgery has been performed (see pages 64 and 74). Staff should evaluate the needs of each person before denying services. Clients who are refused services should be informed again about the availability of vasectomy and temporary methods of contraception, and about the possibility of female sterilization at a later date.

Clients who change their mind before surgery

Every client must understand that she can change her mind about being sterilized—right up to the moment when the fallopian tubes are occluded if she is to be awake during the procedure, or until sedation and general anaesthesia are administered if she is to be asleep. If a client does change her mind, she should be given counselling about other methods of family planning and reassured that she still has the option to undergo sterilization at a later date.

Adjustment after female sterilization

Despite all precautions, a few clients will change their minds, become dissatisfied, or experience other negative reactions after the surgery, often because of remarriage or the death of a child.

As discussed earlier, service providers can minimize these negative reactions by offering a variety of contraceptive choices and by carefully counselling individuals who are interested in voluntary sterilization. Factors associated with negative reactions after female sterilization should also be assessed at the time of preoperative counselling (see page 64).

Some investigators have reported that postpartum and post-abortion sterilizations are associated with higher rates of dissatisfaction than are interval procedures; however, others have reported no difference in these rates (Liskin et al., 1985; Boring et al., 1988). Although the research evidence is mixed, abortion and childbirth are often difficult times to make decisions about sterilization. While these events may present convenient opportunities for tubal occlusion, their stressful nature may lead clients to make choices hastily or without reflection. Care must therefore be taken to ensure that clients in this category consider their decisions carefully—ideally, well before the time of delivery or abortion.

If a client reacts negatively after female sterilization, the provider should offer counselling and support. Reversal services may be offered if they are available in the country and are a realistic possibility for the client.

Payments and benefits to clients

In some countries clients who undergo sterilization receive payments or benefits. The most common type of payment is intended to reimburse the client for costs associated with choosing sterilization (such as travel expenses or lost wages); such payments are meant to make female sterilization accessible to all who want it. In general, such reimbursement payments are not large enough to induce people to choose sterilization, although they may be sufficient to do so for people at the lowest economic level.

Facing population pressures, some countries have encouraged the use of family planning, including voluntary sterilization, by giving payments, gifts, or benefits as incentives unrelated to incurred costs. Such incentives may compromise voluntary choice. Furthermore, offering incentives implicitly suggests that the service involved is more in the interest of the government than of the client. It is therefore best for clients if incentives are avoided altogether.

If a client is to receive a payment or benefit, the counsellor should carefully examine whether it has served as an inducement. The possibility of postoperative dissatisfaction should be carefully discussed during counselling.

Payments, benefits, and targets for providers

Some services pay health care workers according to the number of clients who use family planning methods. Others measure job performance by the number of clients who are recruited. These policies can affect referral agents, outreach workers, nurses, doctors, and others involved in delivering family planning services. Services may adopt these policies to encourage health care personnel to offer family planning services (particularly when they already have a heavy workload), to compensate them for extra work, or to encourage better job performance. Whatever the reason, these policies mean that service staff benefit directly from clients' decisions to use family planning and they should be avoided altogether to protect clients' right to make a voluntary, informed choice.

In some countries, doctors receive per-case payments for medical and surgical procedures, including vasectomy and tubal occlusion. The amount paid for sterilization is comparable to the amount paid for similar procedures. In these instances, most doctors probably do not try to influence the client to undergo sterilization; thus it is acceptable for them to counsel family planning clients. If sterilization is singled out for special compensation, however, doctors should not have primary responsibility for counselling clients (Neamatalla & Harper, 1990).

8. Preoperative care

Once the counselling process has been completed and the client has given her informed consent for sterilization, a number of additional activities are required prior to surgery. The purpose of these preoperative tasks is to determine the client's fitness to undergo sterilization, to identify any conditions that may increase the risks associated with the procedure and anaesthesia, and to confirm that the client's decision is voluntary and informed. The tasks are as follows:

- taking a medical history,
- performing a physical examination,
- carrying out laboratory tests,
- reviewing informed consent (to confirm client understanding and to ensure proper documentation),
- preparing the client emotionally and physically for surgery and anaesthesia.

For clients undergoing sterilization following delivery or pregnancy termination in the same facility, the first three tasks may already have been performed.

Although the preoperative tasks may be carried out by different staff members, and some (such as medical history, physical examination, and laboratory tests) may take place in other locations, the surgeon is responsible for reviewing each client's case record before starting the operation to ensure that all five tasks have been completed satisfactorily.

Medical screening

Medical history

The client's medical history may be taken by the surgeon or by a trained nonphysician. A standard form and list of questions should be used to ensure that all the necessary information is obtained (see page 190). The history should include details of the client's obstetric experience, including previous pregnancies and their outcome; assessment of the client's suitability for the types of anaesthesia available, including previous experience of anaesthesia; any current medications, allergies, and drug dependence; and past illnesses and other medical conditions, such as pelvic disease, abdominal or pelvic surgery, hypertension, diabetes, anaemia, bleeding disorders, heart disease, respiratory problems, convulsions, psychiatric conditions, and recent infections or trauma. The date of the last menstrual period and recent contraceptive use should be ascertained to ensure that the client is not pregnant. If a staff member other than the surgeon takes the history, the surgeon should review the completed form to determine whether any additional information is required.

Medical indications for female sterilization

In most countries there has been a gradual shift away from offering female sterilization only for medical indications and towards making it available for broader health reasons, including the woman's social well-being and her need for contraception. In almost all countries sterilization is provided for certain health indications, such as ruptured uterus, multiple caesarean sections (usually after three or four), or other serious obstetric or medical problems. Some conditions that increase the health risks associated with pregnancy are multiparity, advanced maternal age, previous obstetric complications, medical conditions that can complicate pregnancy (including heart disease, high blood pressure, diabetes, kidney disease, and anaemia), and previous abortions.

Where health indications are required in order to offer sterilization, it is important to include those that will promote a state of optimal physical, mental, and social well-being, as well as those that avert complications from future high-risk pregnancies and deliveries. Frequently the two are interrelated, so that satisfying the woman's wish to end childbearing will also reduce the likelihood of any medical problems related to an unwanted pregnancy occurring in the future. Medical staff should generally grant a woman's request for sterilization if it will improve or prevent deterioration of her health. In any case, women with medical indications for sterilization should still receive complete counselling about the decision and the procedure (see page 72).

Medical contraindications to female sterilization

There are no absolute permanent contraindications to female sterilization if the woman is at risk of an unwanted pregnancy. The medical considerations consist of weighing the relative risks associated with sterilization against the adverse effects of an unintended pregnancy and against the risks associated with alternative means of contraception.

Acute pelvic infection is an absolute, but temporary, contraindication to sterilization. Such infection should be treated, and the client should be provided with a temporary means of contraception until the infection has cleared. While other conditions may increase the risks associated with female sterilization, they may increase the risks associated with pregnancy even more. These relative contraindications, listed below, must be noted and evaluated (and in some cases treated or controlled) before the procedure is carried out:

- a systemic or localized infection
- heart disease
- irregular pulse
- respiratory problems
- hypertension
- mass/lump in the pelvic area
- diabetes
- bleeding disorders
- pregnancy
- severe nutritional deficiencies
- pelvic or abdominal adhesions
- obesity
- umbilical hernia (for laparoscopic and immediate postpartum procedures)

If a medical condition is likely to increase the risks associated with surgery, the client should be either provided with a temporary method of contraception or referred to a better-equipped facility for surgery, if one is available. If both female sterilization and pregnancy pose high risks, the couple should be counselled to consider vasectomy or long-acting temporary contraceptives as alternatives.

Physical examination

A physical examination is part of the preoperative medical screening process. It may be conducted a day or two prior to surgery, or on the day of surgery. If conducted on the day of surgery, however, it should take place before the client has received any premedication, which could mask physical contraindications. This examination should include weighing the woman; checking her temperature, blood pressure, and pulse; auscultation of the heart and lungs; examination of the abdomen; evaluation of the client's nutritional status; checking the skin in the operative area; and other examinations as indicated by the medical history. For clients who have not undergone a recent delivery or abortion, a pelvic examination must also be carried out by the surgeon on the day of the procedure to ensure the absence of infection in the uterus and fallopian tubes; to determine the size, position, and mobility of the uterus; to identify any abnormalities; and to determine the presence or absence of pregnancy.

If surgery is planned on a day-care basis, the client must be instructed to fast on the day of the procedure and to arrange for a family member or friend to look after her during and after her return home.

Temporary contraindications following pregnancy

Several temporary contraindications apply to women who have recently given birth or terminated a pregnancy. If sterilization will increase the risks for these clients, their surgery should be postponed, and they should be given temporary contraception in the interim, if required. These temporary contraindications include the following:

- puerperal sepsis,
- prolonged rupture of membranes (24 hours or more),
- hypertensive states, including pre-eclampsia and eclampsia,
- antepartum or postpartum haemorrhage,
- trauma to the genital tract,
- history of postpartum psychosis.

Another situation that may require postpartum sterilization to be delayed concerns the viability of the newborn (see page 68). This can usually be determined within 10 hours after birth (Pritchard et al., 1985). If the newborn is unhealthy and the child's death might cause the woman to change her mind about sterilization, the procedure should be postponed for a minimum of 6 weeks (42 days). On the other hand, if she does not want any more children, she may wish to go ahead with the procedure even if the baby is not healthy.

Laboratory tests

Laboratory tests can assist in determining whether the surgery should be performed, who should perform it, and where. Tests to screen for anaemia, diabetes, and renal disease (haemoglobin or erythrocyte volume fraction (haematocrit), and urinalysis for sugar and protein) are advisable before all female sterilizations and should be routine if general anaesthesia is to be used. If these tests are not performed on a routine basis at the service site, the surgeon should have access to basic laboratory facilities or to a referral laboratory if he or she suspects any clinical abnormality.

Extensive routine laboratory tests cause unnecessary delays, raise costs, and make very little or no contribution to the quality of care. Accordingly, laboratory testing should be carefully reviewed to avoid conducting unnecessary tests, which may create serious barriers to needed services. In general, additional tests should be avoided unless indicated by the medical history or physical examination. If staff suspect that the woman may be pregnant, a standard pregnancy test should be carried out wherever possible. During the early stages of pregnancy, however, this test may be negative.

For postpartum or postabortion sterilizations, results of basic laboratory tests may be available from the maternity record. The surgeon should check these and reassess the client's haemoglobin level if bleeding was recorded during or immediately after delivery or pregnancy termination.

The clinical staff in each sterilization service should determine the levels of haemoglobin or erythrocyte volume fraction (haematocrit) that require a clinical review. They should also decide whether any clients with anaemia are likely to be vulnerable to cardiovascular complications, especially if general or regional anaesthesia is to be used.

Reviewing informed consent

The operating surgeon must ensure that clients have made voluntary, well-informed decisions and that they understand the sterilization procedure and the type of anaesthesia to be used. In many sterilization services counselling and informed-consent procedures may take place well in advance of surgery and at a different location. The surgeon may not have met or examined the client before the day of the procedure and may not have been responsible for counselling her or for obtaining her consent. Accordingly, the surgeon should review the client records and the informed-consent forms before surgery, as well as talk to staff and at least those clients whom the surgeon believes may have made uninformed, involuntary or poorly considered decisions (see page 64).

This assessment should take place immediately before surgery, and before the client receives any premedication. The client must understand that the procedure is intended to be permanent and must be informed of her right to change her mind or to postpone the operation. This interaction between the surgeon and client can be a valuable opportunity to allay fears and reduce any anxiety the client may have about undergoing surgery.

Preparation of the client before she enters the operating theatre

Physical preparation

On the day of surgery, a staff member should review the pre-operative instructions for physical preparation with the client. These instructions are usually given at an earlier appointment (see page 183). This review should determine whether the client has followed instructions about fasting and bathing before surgery, and whether she has arranged for a friend or family member to escort her home after the operation. Staff should know what to do if the client has not followed these instructions.

Before entering the operating theatre, the client should remove personal effects such as jewellery, hairpins, spectacles, contact lenses, and dentures. This property should be stored in a safe place. The client should also be given a clean gown to wear for the operation.

Shaving or clipping of hair at the operative site is optional. If hair obstructs the area, it should be removed. Clipping is preferable to shaving to reduce the risk of infection. Whichever method is chosen, hair removal should be done immediately before the client is taken into theatre. The client should empty her bladder just before going into theatre.

Emotional preparation

Either the surgeon or another member of staff, preferably a member of the operating team, can serve the important role of preparing the client emotionally for the sterilization procedure. The person responsible should be sensitive to the client's individual needs for reassurance. Opportunities to conduct this activity can be made either during the surgeon's review of informed consent or in conjunction with the physical preparation of the client. This step should allow time to alleviate any concern or fears the client has about the surgery and to answer any last-minute questions. If carried out by the surgeon or by another member of the operating team, this step helps to establish a rapport with the woman before surgery and produces a more relaxed patient, which is especially important if local anaesthesia is to be used.

Clients should not be taken into the operating theatre until the team is ready to start the procedure. This will help prevent prolonged anxiety and discomfort.

9. Anaesthesia[1]

In administering anaesthesia, as in all other technical aspects of delivering female sterilization services, client safety and satisfaction should be the primary considerations. The purpose of anaesthesia is to relieve the patient from pain and discomfort. Premedication may be administered before the anaesthetic to minimize psychological and emotional distress.

Local, regional, or general anaesthesia can be used during female sterilization procedures. Each of these broad categories of anaesthesia has certain advantages and disadvantages, as well as risks and benefits. Service managers and decision makers must be aware of the various factors that determine what type of anaesthesia is required. These factors include the surgical technique selected; the needs and skills of the surgeon and of the anaesthetist (if included in the team); the safety, comfort, and preference of the client; the availability of appropriate drugs; and the ease of managing any complications that may occur.

Types of anaesthesia

Local anaesthesia

Infiltrating a local anaesthetic solution into the operative site causes a loss of sensation in one part of the body. Although some surgeons use only local anaesthesia of the operative site for female sterilization, most augment it with light sedation and mild systemic analgesia.

Under light sedation, the patient is fully responsive, appears awake, and is able to converse coherently but will sleep lightly if unstimulated; this condition should be the goal when sedatives and analgesics are used for female sterilization. Table 13 provides

---

[1] Adapted from *Safe and voluntary surgical contraception*, published by the World Federation of Health Agencies for the Advancement of Voluntary Surgical Contraception, 1988.

Table 13. Comparison of light and heavy sedation with local anaesthesia regimens for female sterilization

Characteristic	Level of sedation	
	Light sedation	Heavy sedation
1. Recommended narcotic dose for 50 kg-woman	Pethidine (meperidine) 50 mg intravenously (and diazepam 10 mg orally)	Pethidine (meperidine) 100 mg intravenously (and diazepam 10 mg orally)
2. Overall level of risk	Low	Moderate (see 7 and 8 below)
3. Relief of pain (analgesia)	Effective, especially with good preoperative counselling and preparation	Is usually more effective during surgery, but may cause more problems and side-effects later
4. Usual conditions of use	Routine, uncomplicated procedure with skilled surgeon and well-trained team using effective local anaesthesia and direct communication with client	For training relatively inexperienced surgeons, for clients specially sensitive to pain, and for difficult or prolonged procedures
5. Level of consciousness	Client fully responsive, appears awake, and is able to converse coherently during procedure; if unstimulated will sleep lightly, but can be aroused with minimal stimulus	Client converses with difficulty, readily falls into deep sleep if unstimulated, and requires vigorous stimulus to arouse
6. Client cooperation during procedure	Client can readily cooperate	Client often unable to cooperate
7. Adverse effects of drugs	Minimal respiratory or cardiovascular depression, which rarely requires ventilatory assistance and reversal of narcotic effects by naloxone; nausea and vomiting infrequent	Moderate respiratory or cardiovascular depression, which occasionally requires ventilatory assistance and reversal of narcotic effects; some patients enter first stage of anaesthesia with delirium, agitation, and noncooperation; nausea and vomiting relatively common

Table 13. (contd)

Characteristic	Level of sedation	
	Light sedation	Heavy sedation
8. Postoperative recovery	Client fully awake and ready to take light snack within 40–60 minutes after surgery	Client usually fully awake within 2–4 hours; requires more frequent and prolonged monitoring of vital signs

a comparison of light and heavy sedation, indicating the advantages of the former. Using local anaesthesia in conjunction with light sedation does not require an anaesthetist, additional personnel or special anaesthetic equipment; however, resuscitation equipment and personnel trained in its use should be available in the event of an emergency. The surgeon and surgical assistant must also be trained in the use of local anaesthesia with light sedation and a refined surgical technique compatible with it.

General anaesthesia

Administering a general anaesthetic intravenously or by inhalation produces or maintains a state of unconsciousness. An anaesthetist (someone trained to administer anaesthesia, not necessarily a doctor) and special equipment are required for procedures using this type of anaesthesia.

Regional anaesthesia

Regional (spinal or epidural) anaesthesia causes the loss of the sensation of pain in a specific region of the body; this effect is produced and maintained by injecting a local anaesthetic solution into the spinal fluid or epidural space of the spinal column. This procedure requires a well-trained anaesthetist. Furthermore, the woman must remain flat during the recovery period following spinal anaesthesia (which is longer than for local anaesthesia) to prevent the occurrence of headache (caused by the loss of cerebrospinal fluid from the brain through the dural puncture).

Method of choice for standardization and safety

Because surgical skills and the quality of facilities may vary, each female sterilization service should use a type of anaesthesia that can be safely administered by available staff and that is appropriate to the surgical setting. Table 14 provides a summary of the comparative advantages and disadvantages of each type of anaesthesia used for female sterilization, together with indications and contraindications for use.

Local anaesthesia with light sedation is generally considered to be the most appropriate technique to employ for female sterilization. Results from large-scale programmes conducted in developing countries indicate that this technique is both safe and cost-effective. It is associated with extremely low rates of morbidity and mortality for both minilaparotomy and laparoscopy (Peterson el al., 1983), as well as a significantly lower risk of complications compared with general and regional anaesthesia. For example, in a sterilization programme conducted in India, in which about 32 000 women were sterilized in 13 teaching hospitals, the complication rates with general, spinal and local anaesthesia were 0.2%, 0.1% and 0.02% respectively (Indian Council of Medical Research, 1982). In addition, local anaesthesia with light sedation is less expensive than the other forms of anaesthesia (although some short-acting general anaesthetic techniques may require less staff time for preoperative discussion with the client and shorter operating times), and it can be readily used in simple settings. As this technique was recommended by a WHO Expert Group on Female Sterilization, local anaesthesia with light sedation will be the focus of the balance of this chapter.[1]

Irrespective of the type of anaesthesia used, it is essential that facilities be available for maintaining a clear airway, including an effective suction machine (which should be tested beforehand), a pharyngeal airway, a laryngoscope and endotracheal tubes, a means of providing artificial ventilation of the lungs in the event of respiratory arrest (for example, with an ambu-bag and mask), and the necessary equipment for setting up an intravenous infusion. Whenever possible, anaesthesia should be deferred for at least 4 hours from the time the patient last ingested either solids

[1] For additional information about regional and general anaesthetic regimens used for female sterilization, see Darney, 1987; Dobson, 1988; Fishburne, 1983; and WFHAAVSC, 1988.

Table 14. Advantages, disadvantages, indications, and contraindications for local, general, and regional anaesthesia for tubal occlusion

	Local anaesthesia with or without sedation	General anaesthesia	Regional anaesthesia
Advantages	Avoids risks of general and regional anaesthesia Low cost Rapid recovery when light or no sedation used Rapid induction Client awake and able to give early warning of some complications Decreased postoperative nausea and vomiting Presence of anaesthetist not required	Complete analgesia Amnesia present Anxiety eliminated	Client awake and able to give early warning of some complications Reduced need for sedation Decreased postoperative nausea and vomiting
Disadvantages	Requires precise and gentle surgical technique Mild to moderate client discomfort Toxicity of local anaesthetic agents	Higher risk to client than local anaesthesia More costly than local anaesthesia; requires an anaesthetist, special equipment and facilities Longer recovery time May cause greater post-operative discomfort Nausea and vomiting common Toxicity of anaesthetic agents	Higher risk to client than local anaesthesia Not easy to administer, requires an anaesthetist with specialized training Takes relatively long time to administer (10–30 minutes for epidural) Recovery slower than with local anaesthesia Toxicity of anaesthetic agents

Indications	All clients without contra-indications for local Setting other than operating theatre Client's fear of general anaesthesia Pulmonary disease Cardiac disease	Anxious client Anticipated difficult procedure	Client's fear of general anaesthesia Pulmonary disease
Contra-indications	Anxious client Conditions increasing operating time and abdominal manipulation of organs (e.g., obesity, pelvic pathology) Sensitivity to intended medications	Severe cardiac or pulmonary disease Client's fear of general anaesthesia Lack of appropriate equipment Sensitivity to intended medications Obesity Inexperienced anaesthetist	Seldom justified for short sterilization procedure Pre-existing back disorder (relative contraindication) Sensitivity to intended medications History of neurological disease Coagulopathy Inexperienced anaesthetist Anxious client Cutaneous infection at injection site Hypovolaemia, severe uncorrected anaemia or cardiac disease

Source: Adapted from WFHAAVSC, 1988, and Fishburne & Keith, 1977.

or liquids. Since trauma significantly delays gastric emptying time, regurgitation or vomiting may still occur even when this rule is observed.

Considerations in the use of local anaesthesia

Because the client is conscious during local anaesthesia, consideration should be given to the following aspects of the procedure: preparation and screening of clients, communication with the client during surgery, and the skill of the operating surgeon and team.

Preparation and screening of clients

Preoperative instruction and preparation are extremely important to ensure the cooperation of the client during the procedure and to keep any fears she may have to a minimum. Further details of these two activities are given on pages 71 and 82. Extreme anxiety about the surgery or about being conscious during the procedure is a contraindication to the use of local or regional anaesthesia. During the preoperative preparation and screening process, staff should discuss the client's emotional state with her and attempt to alleviate any concerns she may have. If the client remains anxious about the procedure, she should be given general anaesthesia if available or referred to a facility where it is available.

Communication during surgery

Because a conscious client is able to monitor the effects of analgesia and often has an early awareness of complications, the surgeon or another member of the surgical team should talk with the client frequently during the procedure. This assists in relaxing the client and helps the surgical team to monitor the effects of the various drugs used.

Skill of the surgeon

Before proceeding with the operation the surgeon must allow time for analgesia and anaesthesia to take effect. Gentle handling of tissues throughout the procedure is important to prevent discomfort and keep the client cooperative. The surgeon must be skilled in performing minilaparotomy or laparoscopy in order to complete the procedure within 15–20 minutes (for simple cases), since many of the analgesics and the effects of local anaesthesia begin to wear off after 30 minutes; this also maintains the confidence of both the client and the surgeon, thus promoting a high level of client satisfaction.

Technique for local anaesthesia

Local anaesthesia with light sedation is generally sufficient to minimize pain and maintain a high level of safety by not compromising the normal physiological control of vital functions. High doses of opioid (narcotic) analgesics and benzodiazepine (tranquillizer) sedatives will compromise respiration, sometimes dramatically, and may cause cardiovascular depression. Therefore, great care is needed to determine the appropriate dosages of these drugs. A sample regimen for use with minilaparotomy is presented below. This is also suitable for laparoscopy, with some modifications, which are noted. All doses given are for an adult weighing 50 kg.

Preoperative medication

Premedication is given to reduce the client's fear and anxiety about surgery. If given orally, it should be administered in time to take effect before the client enters the operating theatre.

The following regimen is suggested:

Between 30 and 60 minutes prior to surgery, sedate the client with diazepam, 10 mg orally (5 mg for clients weighing less than 35 kg). An alternative is to give diazepam, 5–10 mg intravenously, in the operating theatre. However, intravenous diazepam should only be given by a person thoroughly trained in resuscitation or assisted ventilation, who should be responsible for monitoring the client throughout the procedure.

Atropine, 0.02 mg/kg intramuscularly, and promethazine, 25 mg intramuscularly, may also be given at this time. Midazolam, a new short-acting parenteral benzodiazepine that is more expensive and 3–4 times more potent than diazepam, may be substituted for diazepam. Give midazolam one hour before surgery, 2.5–3 mg intramuscularly (WFHAAVSC, 1988).

Analgesics

Before surgery, with the client on the operating table, analgesics are given intravenously to induce systemic analgesia. Pethidine (meperidine) is the preferred drug, administered intravenously in a dose of 50 mg. Alternatively, fentanyl, 0.05–0.06 mg, pentazocine, 15–20 mg or butorphenol, 1 mg intravenously may be given. Half the dose should be given over a period of 30 seconds so the surgical team can note any possible adverse reactions. If none occur, the remainder of the dose should be administered over a period of 30 seconds. In addition to the drugs mentioned above, ketamine (WHO, 1989c) may also be administered either intravenously or intramuscularly to provide short-lasting anaesthesia when muscular relaxation is not required. Ketamine should be administered at 1–2 mg/kg of body weight by slow intravenous injection over a period of 60 seconds. More rapid administration may result in respiratory depression or apnoea and an enhanced pressor response. A dose of 2 mg/kg produces surgical anaesthesia and profound analgesia within 1–2 minutes which may be expected to last 5 to 10 minutes. Alternatively, the drug may be administered at 6–8 mg/kg by deep intramuscular injection. This dose produces surgical anaesthesia within 3–5 minutes and may be expected to last up to 25 minutes.

To counteract respiratory or circulatory depression induced by sensitivity or overdose of the above drugs, the opioid antagonist naloxone should be administered at 0.2–0.4 mg intravenously repeated, as necessary, at 2-minute intervals to a maximum of 10 mg.

Anaesthesia of the operative site

The success of this technique is dependent on placing an adequate volume of local anaesthetic into the correct site. A sample technique is as follows:

1. Infiltrate the skin and subcutaneous tissues of the operative site with 1% lidocaine 5–7 ml (without epinephrine). Allow 1–3 minutes for the anaesthesia to take effect before incising the skin.
2. Inject 1% lidocaine 3–5 ml into the fascia; incise after 1–3 minutes.
3. Inject 1% lidocaine 3–5 ml into the peritoneum and preperitoneal fascia.

4. After opening the peritoneal cavity, drip 1% lidocaine 3–5 ml on to the fallopian tubes and uterus (Fishburne, 1981; WFHAAVSC, 1984). In laparoscopy this step is omitted if the laparoscope does not permit lidocaine application; alternatively, the drug may be applied through a second site, using a long needle.

If double-puncture laparoscopy is used, both sites should be infiltrated.

The maximum safe dose of lidocaine without epinephrine is 4 mg/kg of body weight. For a woman weighing 50 kg, this is 200 mg, or 20 ml of 1% lidocaine. Alternatively, where it is available, lidocaine with epinephrine (at 5 μg/ml) may be used. This provides better haemostasis of the wound. The maximum safe dose of lidocaine with epinephrine is 7 mg/kg. For a woman weighing 50 kg, this is 350 mg, or 35 ml of 1% lidocaine. If only 2% lidocaine is available, it should be diluted to 1% with normal saline in order to obtain an adequate volume for local infiltration without exceeding the safe dose.

Monitoring vital signs

The drugs used for sedation, analgesia, and local anaesthesia may cause changes in breathing, heart rate, blood pressure, or mental functioning. Therefore, monitoring of the client's vital signs must be part of routine practice for all female sterilization procedures, regardless of the anaesthetic and surgical techniques used. All staff should be trained in how to monitor clients who are under the effect of sedation or anaesthesia. This training should include recognizing normal and abnormal drug reactions, determining the physiological baseline for each client, and interpreting changes in the client's condition.

It is essential that monitoring be done before, during, and after the surgical procedure. Staff should measure and record the client's blood pressure, pulse, and respiratory rate, both before and shortly after administering the preoperative sedative. These readings provide a baseline measurement for the client.

During surgery, one member of the medical team should be assigned to monitor and record blood pressure, pulse, and respiratory rate at least once every five minutes. In addition, team members should converse with the client throughout the procedure to assess the effectiveness of local anaesthetic and analgesic drugs.

Following surgery, staff should observe the client continuously, and should measure and record the same vital signs at least once every 15 minutes until they have stabilized at preoperative levels. The client should not be left alone during this period. She should be lying on her side, and staff should be alert to signs of possible distress, such as excessive somnolence, slow respiration (less than 10 breaths per minute—a moderately frequent reaction to heavy sedation), hypotension (systolic blood pressure less than 90 mm Hg), hyperventilation, weak pulse or pulse rate over 90, pallor, or cyanosis. Once the vital signs have stabilized, staff should monitor them every hour until the client is fully awake.

Complications and emergency preparedness

The major complications that may occur with local anaesthesia for both minilaparotomy and laparoscopy are: excessive drug-induced sedation and narcosis, which may produce cardiovascular and respiratory depression (and, if untreated, may lead to cardiorespiratory arrest); toxicity due to drug overdose; and allergic reactions to the anaesthetic (Fishburne, 1983). Allergic reactions are rare if lidocaine is used. These complications are usually caused by improper administration of drugs or inadequate monitoring. Successful management of anaesthesia-induced complications depends on early identification and prompt action. Thus, facilities and equipment for resuscitation should be readily available at all times. Specific measures to take in cases of respiratory and cardiovascular complications, two of the most common complications of anaesthesia, are outlined below.

Respiratory complications

The following actions are recommended for the management of respiratory complications associated with anaesthesia.

- Keep the airway open.
- Oxygenate the patient using resuscitation equipment.
- Check the circulation by monitoring pulse, blood pressure, and respiratory rate.

- If an opiate drug has been used, administer naloxone[1] 0.2–0.4 mg intravenously. Repeat this dose within 2–3 minutes if the desired improvement in respiratory function is not obtained.
- If the client has aspirated gastric contents, apply suction to the trachea immediately and begin treatment as indicated. Monitor the client carefully for signs of adult respiratory distress syndrome, the onset of which may be delayed by 12–24 hours.

Cardiovascular complications

To prevent cardiovascular complications, sedatives should be given slowly, with close monitoring of the client's vital signs. The dose must be adjusted according to the client's body weight and general health condition.

If serious cardiovascular complications occur, the surgical team should be prepared to provide basic cardiopulmonary resuscitation[2] as follows.

- If cardiac arrest is confirmed, give an immediate precordial thump and begin external cardiac massage.
- In the case of respiratory arrest, give 100% oxygen through resuscitation equipment (or begin mouth-to-mouth resuscitation).
- Cannulate a vein and administer resuscitative drugs as appropriate. The following common drugs may be used: naloxone (as above), epinephrine, lidocaine, atropine, and sodium bicarbonate solution. (This list is illustrative only and is not intended to be complete.)

---

[1] Naloxone should be the drug of choice for respiratory depression when narcotics have been used. It does not reverse the effects of ketamine. It acts promptly, has little toxicity, and is quickly metabolized. Staff must monitor the client closely during its use because the effect of the narcotic causing the depression may outlast the effect of naloxone. Repeat administration of naloxone may be required. Several doses given over a short period usually have no adverse effects. If naloxone 0.2–0.4 mg produces no response, staff must consider other causes of respiratory depression, such as overdose of diazepam or hypoxic central nervous system injury. Toxicity due to diazepam can be treated with physostigmine 0.5–1.0 mg intravenously.

[2] For more information on cardiopulmonary resuscitation, see Dobson, 1988, and King, 1986.

Emergency preparedness

The resuscitation and emergency equipment required to deal with complications of anaesthesia is indicated on page 145. All the necessary equipment for emergency resuscitation must be readily available whenever anaesthesia or sedation is planned in the operating theatre and accessible to the recovery area, and should be sterilized, prepared for use, and in good working order. Staff should be familiar with its use and should check all items before each operating session.

If possible, services should have a physician or anaesthetist on the staff who has been trained in intubation and the use of a laryngoscope. An anaesthetist to administer general anaesthesia is particularly appropriate where laparoscopy is used. Where such trained personnel are available, a laryngoscope and a set of endotracheal tubes should be on hand for every female sterilization procedure. If personnel have not been trained in intubation or if they do not practise these skills regularly, oral or nasopharyngeal airways and manual resuscitators with face masks are the preferred means of ventilation.

10. Surgery

This chapter will discuss primarily the surgical techniques described briefly in Chapter 2. Although relatively simple, the surgery for female sterilization requires meticulous attention to detail in order to ensure safety and client satisfaction with the procedure. In particular, a strict aseptic technique must be employed and maintained throughout the procedure, and the surgical team must be well trained in the selection and use of appropriate surgical techniques (see Chapter 2).

Aseptic technique

As infection is one of the major risks and complications of female sterilization, strict attention to aseptic technique is mandatory in all female sterilization services and is required at all times—before, during, and after surgery. Aseptic technique should be stressed in training and in monitoring and supervision of medical services. The principles of asepsis as they apply to staff, clients, and surgery are discussed below. Recommended methods for the sterilization and disinfection of facilities, equipment, and instruments are discussed on page 137.

Personnel

Any personnel who have an infection should not be allowed in the operating theatre. Movement into and out of the operating theatre should be minimized. Before entering the operating theatre, all personnel should put on a clean surgical scrub suit and gown, a mask to cover the mouth and nose, a cap to cover all the hair on the head and face, and a clean pair of shoes or shoe-covers.

All members of the surgical team should also complete a surgical scrub using soap and water or antiseptic agents containing hexachlorophene, chlorhexidine, or an iodine preparation (e.g., povidone–iodine). A brush should be used on the nails and fingertips. Ethanol (70% by volume) may be used to rinse the hands after the surgical scrub; this procedure is recommended for facilities where surgical scrubbing is done with soap and water only (Porter, 1987).

After scrubbing their hands and drying them, all members of the surgical team should put on sterile gloves. The gloves must be changed between cases. Whenever a glove is punctured during a procedure it should also be promptly changed. Ideally, the surgeon and surgical assistant should scrub thoroughly before each case. In high-volume settings, this may not be feasible because the skin cannot tolerate the irritation caused by frequent scrubbing. In these situations, the surgical team should scrub for three minutes every hour or after every four or five cases (whichever comes first), to prevent recolonization of the skin by microorganisms. They should scrub and change gowns after every infected case and if they leave the operating theatre for any reason. Team members should also scrub whenever gloves are torn.

Clients

The operative site should be prepared immediately before surgery with an antiseptic solution such as 2.5% iodine in alcohol (25 g/litre), povidone–iodine, or chlorhexidine. The umbilicus should be thoroughly cleansed for laparoscopy and periumbilical postpartum minilaparotomy procedures. For interval minilaparotomy and laparoscopy procedures, the surgeon should cleanse the vagina and cervix with an antiseptic before inserting the uterine manipulator. Alcohol preparations should not be applied to the genitalia.

Surgery

Use of a gentle surgical technique minimizes the degree of tissue trauma. Minimizing bleeding and checking to ensure there is no bleeding at closure will reduce the risk of haematoma, as well as the likelihood and severity of infection (see also pages 113 and 115).

Postpartum procedures

The period immediately following vaginal delivery is the most common time for performing female sterilization in many countries. Many services schedule sterilization procedures 10 hours or more after delivery; this allows sufficient time to assess the condition of the baby and, in most cases, to identify women who will have postpartum haemorrhage (Pritchard et al., 1985). Postpartum procedures should be performed within 48 hours of delivery if possible. In general, postpartum procedures are more convenient for the client, less costly, and easier to perform than procedures done at other times; they may also make use of existing facilities and personnel. A simple minilaparotomy procedure performed within 48 hours of delivery does not extend the normal postdelivery hospital stay. In all cases of postpartum or postabortion sterilization, counselling and informed-consent procedures should be completed well in advance of the delivery or termination, if possible (see pages 61 and 69).

After 48 hours, the uterus becomes less accessible, and a slightly larger and lower incision is therefore necessary. Consequently, while female sterilization may be performed 3–7 days postpartum, it is slightly more difficult at this time. Also, because bacteria from the vagina may have ascended into the tubes and uterine cavity by this time, medical personnel should consider giving prophylactic antibiotics (Wheeless & Katayama, 1985). If sterilization is not performed within 7 days of delivery, it should be delayed until after 6 weeks (42 days) postdelivery, when the uterus has returned to its normal size and position. An interval (suprapubic) minilaparotomy can then be performed, using the uterine manipulator and without prophylactic antibiotics (see also pages 14 and 20). After 6 weeks (42 days) following delivery, however, the risk of becoming pregnant again begins to increase for women who are not fully breast-feeding. Therefore, they should be given temporary contraception to use until the sterilization (Darney, 1987). For fully breast-feeding, amenorrhoeic women, contraception may be delayed until 4–6 months postdelivery with a relatively low risk of pregnancy. However, as soon as a woman starts to supplement her infant's feeding, she should begin using contraception.

Female sterilization may also be performed in conjunction with first-trimester spontaneous or induced abortion, or at the time of caesarean section; however, in no case should it be a reason for undergoing caesarean delivery, nor should pregnancy termination be carried out on the condition that the woman undergoes a sterilization.

Surgical approach

After delivery, when the uterus is high in the abdomen (see Fig. 6), a small minilaparotomy incision (3–4 cm) just below the top of the fundus, which is approximately at the level of the umbilicus, is usually adequate to reach the tubes. The procedure is performed with the woman in the supine position. It should be ensured that her bladder is empty (catheterizing if necessary) before starting the procedure. Local anaesthesia, alone or in conjunction with light sedation and analgesia (as described on page 91), is usually sufficient, because several of the more painful aspects of minilaparotomy—the bimanual examination, use of the lithotomy position, application of the cervical tenaculum, and use of the uterine manipulator—are usually unnecessary in

Fig. 6. The uterus and fallopian tubes after delivery

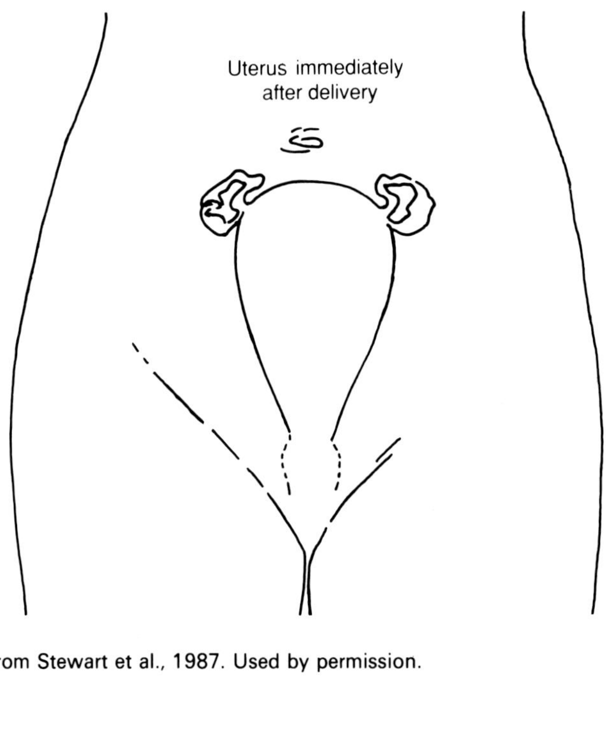

Adapted from Stewart et al., 1987. Used by permission.

postpartum procedures. Furthermore, postpartum minilaparotomy requires a smaller incision than interval minilaparotomy. The tubes can be reached easily by moving the incision site in the loose abdominal wall over each tube or by moving the uterus by pressing a hand against the side of the abdomen.

If minilaparotomy is not feasible, laparotomy (involving an abdominal incision of more than 5 cm) may be performed. This procedure usually requires hospitalization, the use of heavy sedation, general anaesthesia, or regional anaesthesia. The longer incision and additional anaesthesia requirements increase the risks associated with the procedure and prolong the recovery time. However, the technique is used when sterilization is performed in conjunction with caesarean section, since the incision required for delivery allows immediate access to the tubes.

Laparoscopy should not be performed in the postpartum period because of the possibility of injury to the large, vascular uterus. However, this approach may be used following first-trimester abortion. The alternative postabortion approach is similar to the interval minilaparotomy, as described on page 102. In this case, however, the incision is slightly higher than the suprapubic incision indicated in Fig. 7, and a uterine manipulator is not used.

Occlusive techniques

Several recommended surgical occlusive techniques used for female sterilization are illustrated in Fig. 2 (page 18); their main features are summarized in Tables 4 and 5 (pages 15 and 19). The Pomeroy technique, using plain catgut, is a widely used method of tubal occlusion and has proven to be effective and safe in the postpartum period.

The Parkland technique is another effective method of ligation and resection, in which chromic catgut is used to occlude the tubes. This technique is also commonly used for postpartum sterilization procedures (Liskin et al., 1985; Pritchard et al., 1985). The technique avoids approximation of the cut ends, which can lead to failures, and preserves more of the tube and adjacent blood vessels than the Pomeroy technique. Some surgeons believe preservation of these vessels may help prevent future pelvic congestion and altered ovarian function. However, whether other occlusive techniques cause these conditions is uncertain. Surgeons who wish to maximize the possibility of reversal may use the Parkland technique, removing a small (1–2 cm) segment from the isthmic portion of the tube.

Fimbriectomy has been associated with high rates of failure and more postoperative complications than either the Pomeroy or Parkland technique and, therefore, should not be used.

Various mechanical methods may also be used to achieve tubal occlusion. The Filshie clip is suitable for use in postpartum procedures, as it can accommodate the enlarged postpartum fallopian tube. However, the surgeon must apply the clip carefully and slowly, to squeeze out any excess fluid in the tube and to ensure that the clip closes completely over the tube. The clip should be applied 1–2 cm from the uterus. The silicone band and the spring clip are less suitable for immediate postpartum application, as they may not accommodate the enlarged tube.

At caesarean section, the Pomeroy, Parkland, and Irving are the most commonly recommended occlusive techniques. The Irving technique requires a wide surgical field, which is possible in connection with caesarean deliveries, and is one of the most effective methods of occlusion. However, the Irving technique is not widely used as it takes a relatively long time to perform. The Filshie clip may also be used for these procedures, and should be applied as described above.

The fallopian tubes are usually less engorged and oedematous after abortion than immediately following a term delivery, but they should still be handled carefully, regardless of the occlusive technique selected. The Pomeroy and Parkland procedures are most suitable for postabortion minilaparotomies; silicone bands and Filshie clips have been used satisfactorily with laparoscopy procedures performed at this time.

Interval procedures

Surgical approach

Suprapubic minilaparotomy is a widely used technique for interval female sterilization (performed 6 weeks (42 days) or more after delivery). Minilaparotomy may be difficult if the woman is obese or if she has tubal adhesions from infection or previous surgery. When a uterine manipulator is used, the woman is usually placed in the lithotomy position but she may be supine. After checking to ensure that the client's bladder is empty (catheterizing if necessary), the surgeon performs a pelvic examination (if this was not included at the time of the screening procedure). A cervical tenaculum is usually applied before the uterine manipulator is inserted. The uterine manipulator is then used to bring the fundus of the uterus closer to the abdominal wall. A 3–4 cm abdominal incision is made just above the fundus, usually 3 cm above the pubic hairline (symphysis pubis) (see Fig. 7). Correct placement of the incision is essential to avoid injuring the bladder and to allow the surgeon to reach the tubes easily. The procedure may also be performed with the woman tilted in the head-down (Trendelenburg) position (not more than 20°). A tubal hook, small Babcock forceps or even the surgeon's fingers are often used to lift the tubes from the abdomen. This is facilitated by moving the uterus with the manipulator to expose each tube. Without use of the manipulator, the tubes may be difficult to reach, especially if the uterus is retroverted (tilted back).

Laparoscopy is another approach often used for interval female sterilization (see Fig. 8). This approach employs a sophisticated instrument containing fibre-optic cylinders that transmit light and allow the surgeon to visualize the abdominal

Fig. 7. Incision site for minilaparotomy female sterilization, interval procedure

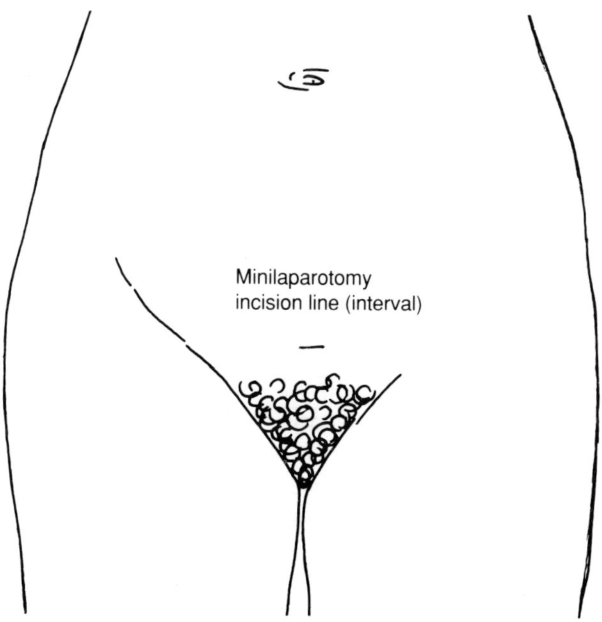

Fig. 8. Laparoscope illuminating the abdominal cavity

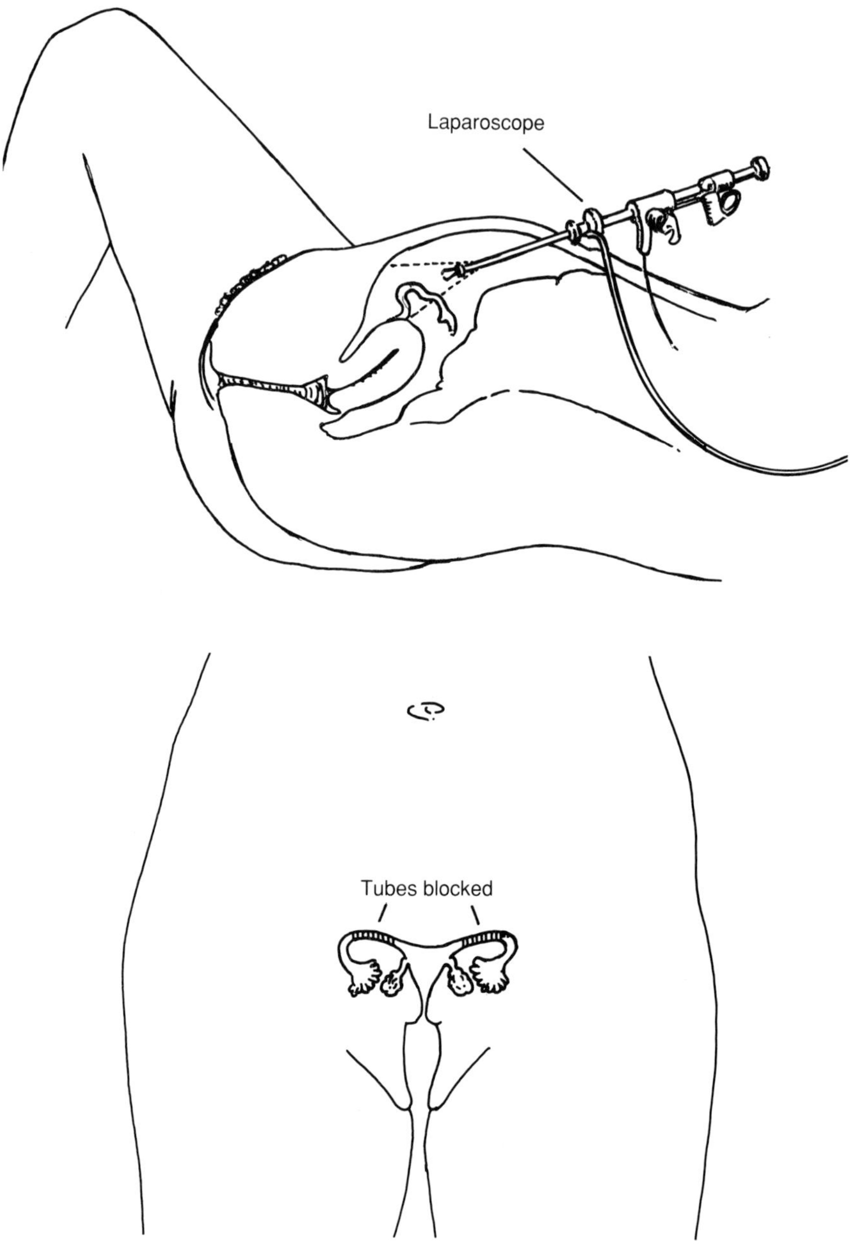

Adapted from Stewart et al., 1987. Used by permission.

cavity. Laparoscopy may be performed using either a single- or a double-puncture technique, in which the surgeon passes the occlusion instrument and the instruments for occluding the tubes through a single channel or two separate channels.

With the client in the Trendelenburg position (no more than 15°), the first step in laparoscopy is to inflate the abdomen with 1–3 litres of gas (carbon dioxide, nitrous oxide, or room air) through a Veress needle placed in a small subumbilical skin incision. The gas separates the abdominal wall from the organs to provide a clear view of the organs and allow safe introduction of the laparoscope. The surgeon removes the needle, enlarges the skin incision, and inserts a trocar with its cannula. The surgeon then removes the trocar and inserts the laparoscope through the cannula. The second puncture, if used, should be 3 cm above the symphysis in the midline, or just adjacent to the midline under direct vision through the laparoscope (Liskin et al., 1985).

A variation of this technique–open laparoscopy–involves making a subumbilical incision similar to that for postpartum minilaparotomy before placing a cannula (with a blunt obturator) and then inserting the laparoscope. This procedure may reduce the risk of injury to the bowel or blood vessels associated with closed (conventional) laparoscopy during "blind" entry of the insufflation needle and trocar (Hasson, 1984, 1982; Penfield, 1980).

Occlusive techniques

For interval minilaparotomy procedures, the Pomeroy and Parkland ligation and resection techniques are appropriate, as are silicone bands, Filshie clips, and spring clips (see Table 4). Fimbriectomy has been associated with higher failure rates than these techniques, provides no advantages over them, and usually cannot be reversed. The Irving technique cannot be performed through a minilaparotomy incision.

Silicone bands, Filshie clips, and spring clips are usually applied by laparoscopy. Silicone bands should be placed 3 cm from the uterus, and clips at 1–2 cm (see Fig. 2, page 18). The fallopian tube must be carefully identified to avoid placing these devices on the round ligament. It is essential that the clips are placed across the entire tube. The spring clip, having a lower force of compression than the Filshie clip, requires special care to avoid failure. The spring clip should be placed at a 90° angle across the tube, with the isthmic portion of the tube positioned at the hinged part of the jaws. This precision may be difficult to achieve except by very experienced laparoscopists.

Electrocoagulation, either unipolar or bipolar, may be performed by laparoscopy. However, the risk of ectopic pregnancy reported with either method of electrocoagulation is higher than that associated with bands or clips (Kwak, 1987; Whong, 1987). Burns to the bowel, bladder, and abdominal wall may also occur (see page 20).

Completing the procedure

For minilaparotomy and open laparoscopy procedures, it is unnecessary for the surgeon to suture the peritoneum afterwards, because the defect will heal naturally without increased risk of adhesions (Callaghan, 1986; Hasson, 1984; McFadden & Peacock, 1983). However, the abdominal wound should be closed in layers, and the skin closed with absorbable or nonabsorbable sutures. The wound should then be covered with an adhesive bandage.

Other surgical approaches

Vaginal approaches

The fallopian tubes can be reached, drawn down, and occluded through an incision high in the vagina behind the cervix, either by direct visualization (colpotomy) or by use of an operating scope (culdoscopy). These techniques are difficult to learn and perform, and they have been associated with relatively high rates of infection, pain, surgical accidents, and failure. Therefore, vaginal approaches are not recommended for general use (WFHAAVSC, 1988).

Transcervical approaches

These largely experimental techniques may utilize an operating scope (hysteroscope) inserted through the cervix to visualize the ostia of the fallopian tubes. Various occlusive materials, such as silicone rubber, can be injected into the tubes through this instrument. These techniques are difficult to perform, the equipment is expensive, and the success rates are generally poor. Accordingly, they should not be used on a routine basis. Simpler techniques without direct visualization of the tubal openings have been used to introduce chemicals into the tubes or uterine cavity, but the rates of successful occlusion, at least with one application, are not yet comparable with those associated with abdominal surgical approaches (Zatuchni et al., 1983).

Hysterectomy

The removal of the uterus makes a woman sterile, but this should never be done solely for sterilization purposes. Hysterectomy is an extensive surgical procedure and should be performed only for medical indications, separate from the contraceptive rationale.

11. Postoperative care

Postoperative care includes care immediately after surgery, assessment of recovery before discharge, postoperative instruction, follow-up examination if applicable, and detection and management of any complications.

Postoperative monitoring[1]

Responsibility for monitoring does not end with the transfer of the client from the operating theatre to the recovery area. After surgery, staff should be assigned to observe the client, and to monitor her blood pressure, pulse, and respiratory rate every 15 minutes until they have stabilized at preoperative levels. Thereafter, vital signs should be monitored every hour until the client has fully recovered from the effects of anaesthesia. When the client has recovered, she should be able to dress herself and should not sway or fall when standing with her feet close together and her eyes closed (Romberg's test). As soon as she feels able to take something by mouth, she should be given liquids and bland carbohydrates to raise her blood sugar and carbohydrate levels. The client may be discharged when she does not have excessive pain and she is able to dress herself and to converse coherently. She should be accompanied home by a responsible adult.

Postoperative instructions

When the client is fully awake, and before she is discharged, a trained staff member should review with her all instructions related to postoperative concerns and care. Since it may be difficult

[1] See also page 93.

for the woman to remember instructions given at this time, it is important that they were thoroughly reviewed before surgery, that a family member or a close friend is included in the review, and that written instructions are also given (see page 71). A sample set of postoperative instructions is provided in Annex 2. Service staff should ensure that the client is fully informed about:

- how to care for the wound,
- how to use any postoperative medications that are prescribed,
- how to recognize signs of complications and what to do if they occur (see Chapter 12),
- when to resume normal activities,
- when and where to go for the follow-up visit.

The client should be given an opportunity to ask questions about the instructions and discuss any concerns she may have.

Written instructions are especially important if the woman develops a serious complication. This information may then be life-saving. She must know which problems require her to go to a health care facility immediately. She should also know how to reach the nearest clinic or hospital with staff who are able to recognize and treat complications associated with tubal occlusion.

Most otherwise healthy women who undergo an interval sterilization should be able to resume normal activities within 3–5 days of surgery. For healthy women undergoing routine sterilization in connection with a delivery or termination of pregnancy, the sterilization should not extend the usual associated period of hospitalization or rest. To minimize the risk of thromboembolism associated with prolonged bed rest postpartum, it is important to adopt a small-incision minilaparotomy technique, which can be done with local anaesthesia, causes few side-effects, and leads to rapid postoperative recovery.

Follow-up

Postsurgery examination

Ideally, a follow-up examination should be conducted 7 days after surgery, and in any event not later than 2 weeks after the procedure. The use of nonabsorbable sutures to close the skin incision increases the likelihood that the client will return for a follow-up examination, because she will need to have the stitches removed. However, nonabsorbable sutures increase the risk of infection if they are not removed within 7 days.

The operating surgeon should conduct the follow-up examination if possible. However, in some cases it may be more convenient for another member of the medical team to examine the client or for the client to visit another health facility for follow-up. In some settings the follow-up examination is conducted at the client's home. Any trained health professional can conduct this examination, unless the woman has a major complication, in which case she should see a doctor, preferably the operating surgeon. If the follow-up examination takes place at a facility other than the provider site or is conducted by staff other than the surgical team, any complications observed should be reported to the team.

The follow-up visit should include an examination of the operative site, removal of sutures (if nonabsorbable sutures were used), and any other examination or treatment which may be required. If any problems arise that cannot be readily resolved, the health professional should schedule another follow-up visit or refer the client to a higher-level facility.

If a client is referred to another health centre for follow-up or for treatment of complications, she should be given a copy of her medical record or a referral note containing the following information:

- date of procedure,
- type of procedure,
- name of the operating surgeon and facility,
- any special instructions to the person conducting the follow-up examination.

The original record must be maintained at the provider site to ensure accurate service monitoring (see Chapter 18).

During the initial follow-up examination, the staff should be alert to any complaints suggesting that the client is reacting negatively to sterilization. If later follow-up visits are made, staff should try to identify any signs of dissatisfaction, regret, misunderstanding, or maladjustment related to the sterilization. Further counselling or referral should be provided if necessary.

Community follow-up

Negative psychological effects resulting from sterilization may occur much later than the postsurgery follow-up visit. If community field-workers or any other outreach health staff are involved in the service, they should be fully conversant with immediate follow-up instructions, and able to detect later signs of regret, other client concerns, and complications related to sterilization. Community workers are often the health care staff most likely to be aware of changes in a client's life, such as remarriage or loss of a child, that might cause her to regret her decision to be sterilized. They are often the most appropriate people to provide preliminary advice and to refer the client to the service site for additional counselling as required.

12. Complications[1] and side-effects: prevention and management

In general, female sterilization using the techniques described in earlier chapters is a safe procedure, and few women experience complications. This chapter discusses the most common complications and side-effects related to the procedure, according to the point at which they occur or are detected and their severity. For the purpose of this discussion, the following definitions have been applied:

- *Side-effects, or complaints*, are symptoms attributable to the surgery but not requiring exceptional intervention. These include pain in the abdomen, shoulder, or chest, nausea, and vomiting.
- *Complications* are problems directly related to the surgery or the anaesthesia that occur within 42 days and that require intervention and management beyond what would normally be provided. These include infection, bleeding, unintended injury, and depressed respiration or blood pressure due to anaesthesia.

A further distinction is sometimes made between major and minor complications. *Major complications* require hospitalization, surgery, blood transfusion, or treatment of life-threatening events, or result in death (WFHAAVSC, 1983). Most reporting systems include only major complications. *Minor complications* require intervention and management beyond what would normally be provided, but do not progress to any of the five events above.

Complication rates for female sterilization depend to a large extent on the sophistication of the service site and the experience

[1] Complications directly associated with anaesthesia are discussed on page 94. The equipment required to deal with anaesthetic and surgical emergencies is discussed on page 145.

of the surgeons and staff. Reported rates are also influenced by the definition of complications and by the accuracy of reporting. Rates reported from different sites may therefore not be comparable.

Intraoperative complications

The most common types of complications that occur during female sterilization surgery are cardiovascular and respiratory problems related to anaesthesia (see page 94) and problems associated with bleeding. Injury may occur to the uterus (through perforation with the uterine manipulator), bowel, bladder, or other internal organs. Overall, rates of major complications are very low for female sterilization procedures—usually in the range of 0.4–2.0%. The risk of complications during surgery depends on the skill and experience of the surgeon, the characteristics of the client, and the type of procedure and occlusive technique used. Adequate training, surgical skill, and regular practice are important factors in preventing surgical complications. This is especially true for laparoscopy, which is technically a more complicated procedure than minilaparotomy. Clients with a history of abdominal or pelvic surgery are more likely to experience complications, particularly when laparoscopy is used. Other client risk factors are a history of diabetes mellitus or pelvic infection, lung disease, and obesity (DeStefano et al., 1983).

Most intraoperative complications can be prevented or at least reduced to a minimum by proper screening, use of local anaesthesia with light sedation, strict monitoring of vital signs, adherence to strict aseptic technique, and careful surgical technique. The severity of complications can be minimized by early recognition and prompt management.

Preventing complications of postpartum sterilization

Before undertaking postpartum sterilization, providers must rule out postpartum haemorrhage or any condition that would increase the risk of infection or complications of anaesthesia (see page 77). Since the abdominal wall is thin at the umbilicus, the surgeon must take care in making the incision to avoid cutting the intestine. The tissues, fallopian tubes, and mesosalpinx should be handled gently, and ligatures and clips should be applied securely in order to prevent bleeding from the engorged postpartum vessels. These points also apply to the handling of the tubes in the postabortion period. In all minilaparotomy procedures, the surgeon should inspect the tissues carefully before closing the incision, to make sure that there is no bleeding.

As discussed earlier, postpartum procedures are usually performed within 48 hours of delivery to minimize the risk of bacteria ascending into the tubes (see page 99; WFHAAVSC, 1988). Two studies of postpartum minilaparotomy have reported low rates of 0.3% for major complications (Indian Council of Medical Research, 1982; WHO Task Force on Female Sterilization, 1982a).

Preventing complications of interval sterilization

The surgeon must take care to avoid incising the bladder during suprapubic minilaparotomy procedures. This problem can be prevented if the client's bladder is emptied, either by voiding immediately before the operation or by catheterization in the operating theatre. The uterine manipulator must be used gently to avoid perforating the uterus.

Although the frequency of complications related to the use of laparoscopy is similar to that associated with minilaparotomy, some complications of laparoscopy are more severe. The gas-filled abdomen and the use of the Trendelenburg position can aggravate anaesthesia-related complications. Insertion of the insufflation needle or the trocar can cause injuries to blood vessels, intestines, or other organs. In order to avoid these complications, laparoscopy must be performed by specialists, such as obstetrician-gynaecologists, who have been trained in laparoscopy and follow recognized guidelines on safe practice (WFHAAVSC, 1988).

All methods of tubal occlusion require a careful surgical technique to prevent tearing and bleeding of the fallopian tubes and mesosalpinx. Sutures, bands, and clips must be applied carefully and correctly. In some countries where pelvic inflammatory disease and thickened tubes are relatively common, surgeons applying a band with laparoscopy tear the tube in approximately one case in 10. Some centres in these countries are therefore abandoning bands in favour of minilaparotomy using the Pomeroy technique (J. Dwyer, personal communication, 1989).

Early postoperative side-effects and complications

Side-effects

Following surgery, most patients will probably experience some discomfort. After sterilization, generalized lower abdominal pain is common. Women undergoing laparoscopy may experience chest and shoulder pain for one or two days after surgery due to insufflation of the abdomen and incomplete evacuation of gas afterwards. Among the occlusive techniques, silicone bands appear to cause more postoperative pain than other methods. This may be because the nerve endings in the avascular loop of the tube trapped in the band continue to function for several days. Application of local anaesthesia to the tubes during the procedure provides temporary relief. These side-effects may also be relieved by mild analgesics (Liskin et al., 1985). Other side-effects include nausea and vomiting.

Complications

Most major complications related to female sterilization occur at the time of surgery and are related to the anaesthesia (see page 94) or to surgical accidents, as noted above. Occasionally an injury to the internal organs or bleeding that is undetected during surgery will manifest itself as a major, life-threatening complication during the immediate postoperative recovery period or after discharge (sometimes several days later). These complications are largely preventable if strict attention is given to safe technique. Early recognition and prompt treatment of any problems that do occur will minimize their severity. Clear postoperative instructions (written and oral) also encourage the client to return promptly if she has symptoms of a complication (see page 108).

Poststerilization pelvic infection can occur and may be severe if surgery is performed on a fallopian tube that is already infected. A careful pelvic examination is essential before an interval procedure to detect any pre-existing pelvic infection. In these cases, high-dose antibiotic treatment is needed, and a second operation, to remove infected tissue, may be necessary. Although wound infections are usually minor, they may be severe and have occasionally been associated with necrotizing fasciitis (gas gangrene), a very serious condition. Strict asepsis, careful cleaning of the operative site immediately before surgery, and attention to bleeding during surgery to ensure haemostasis can reduce postoperative infection rates. In addition, the client should be given complete instructions on postoperative care of the surgical wound.

Comparison of complication rates for interval minilaparotomy and laparoscopy

In studies where interval minilaparotomy (Pomeroy) and laparoscopy (bands) have been compared, the rates for major complications have generally ranged between 0.4% and 2.0%. However, because some complications of laparoscopy are more severe, most authors conclude that minilaparotomy is the preferred technique except in large, well-equipped institutions (Mumford et al., 1980; WHO Task Force on Female Sterilization, 1982b). The largest reported multicentre study found a surgical complication rate of 0.8% for minilaparotomy Pomeroy procedures and of 2.0% for laparoscopy procedures using bands (Mumford et al., 1980). Another multicentre study in one country found major complication rates of 0.4% for minilaparotomy Pomeroy and 1.2% for laparoscopy (electrocoagulation and band) procedures (Indian Council of Medical Research, 1982).

Mortality

Generally speaking, practising contraception is substantially safer than pregnancy and childbirth. It makes sense, therefore, in terms of health policy, to offer contraceptive services to women. This general consideration, however, should not be the basis for advising individual women that they should use contraception or on what particular kind of contraception they should use. Advice about the risks and benefits of the various options should always be related to the particular circumstances of the client.

Female sterilization may be the safest option for many women when considered in terms of reproductive mortality (deaths related to a contraceptive method as well as deaths due to pregnancies resulting from method failure). The relative safety of the procedure is a result of two special features of the method:

- The risks associated with the sterilization procedure are largely limited to the time of surgery, rather than continuing or increasing over time, as do the risks associated with some other methods.

- Sterilization is almost 100% effective; therefore, the potential risks of additional future pregnancies (contraceptive failures) are extremely low.

In general, the rates of mortality associated with female sterilization reported from developing countries range from 4 to 20 per 100 000 procedures; many rates are less than 10 per 100 000 (Ross et al., 1985). Furthermore, mortality rates are similar for interval minilaparotomy and laparoscopy, as well as for procedures performed immediately after delivery or abortion and interval procedures. By comparison, maternal mortality rates range from 300 to 800 per 100 000 births in most developing countries (Starrs, 1987). Therefore, the risk posed by a single pregnancy is 30–80 times that associated with sterilization (Huber, 1989). And 1.5–2.5 births are averted per sterilization in most countries where estimates have been made (Ross et al., 1985).

In one developing country, where sterilizations were performed using heavy sedation (pethidine 100 mg, plus diazepam 10 mg), the mortality rate was 19 deaths per 100 000 procedures. When protocols were changed to light sedation with closer monitoring of vital signs, this rate declined to 4–8 deaths per 100 000 procedures (Grimes et al., 1982). Reports from over 40 countries show a pattern of declining anaesthesia- and infection-related fatalities from 1973 to 1987. However, surgical injuries, including bowel lacerations with minilaparotomy, declined less rapidly (Huber et al., 1987).

Anaesthesia has been a prominent cause of sterilization-related deaths. General anaesthesia, regional anaesthesia, and heavy sedation have been identified as risk factors. As a result, the World Federation of Health Agencies for the Advancement of Voluntary Surgical Contraception has recommended the widespread use of local anaesthesia with light sedation. Fatalities have also resulted from haemorrhage, sepsis, and, with laparoscopy, insufflation accidents, burns caused by electrocoagulation, and other injuries to internal organs caused by trocar entry.

Long-term side-effects

Menstrual disorders

Studies undertaken to investigate changes in menstrual bleeding after sterilization, including prospective analysis of the duration and quantity of subsequent menses, have generally failed to demonstrate any change in bleeding up to two years following surgery (Liskin et al., 1985). However, many reported changes in menstrual patterns after sterilization appear to be related to the discontinuation of methods of contraception that are known to induce changes in the menstrual pattern, such as oral contraceptives and intrauterine devices. For postpartum clients, observed changes in menstruation may be related to the resumption of normal bleeding patterns following pregnancy. Menstrual bleeding does not appear to be affected by hormonal changes following female sterilization (Hatcher et al., 1988).

Gynaecological problems

Recent well-controlled prospective studies comparing sterilized women with those who have not been sterilized have found, contrary to earlier reports, that the former have no greater risk of hospital referral for uterine prolapse, menstrual disorders, pelvic infections, cervicitis or cervical erosion, hysterectomy, or dilatation and curettage (Vessey et al., 1983).

Often studies that have reported higher rates of hysterectomy and other gynaecological problems following sterilization have not taken sufficient account of pre-existing health problems. Also, sterilized women, having already experienced abdominal surgery, may be less reluctant than others to undergo hysterectomy recommended for subsequent problems; if this is the case, hysterectomy rates for sterilized women would appear inflated (Liskin et al., 1985).

Ectopic pregnancy

Ectopic pregnancy (development of a fertilized egg outside the uterus) is a potentially life-threatening complication resulting from sterilization failure. Overall, the incidence of pregnancy following sterilization is very low (see Table 3, page 12). However, 4–64% of these pregnancies are reported to be ectopic as compared with approximately 1% among women who have not been sterilized. Ectopic pregnancies have been reported as early as two months and as late as eight years after sterilization (DeStefano et al., 1982; Kwak, 1987; Liskin et al., 1985; Whong, 1987).

Although most studies fail to draw any firm conclusions regarding techniques of occlusion to prevent these events, recent studies from the Republic of Korea have found an increased incidence of ectopic pregnancy among women undergoing sterilization by unipolar or bipolar electrocoagulation. As a result, the Government no longer compensates surgeons who use this occlusive technique for sterilization procedures and will not reimburse doctors for treating complications associated with its use (S. V. Kim, personal communication, 1987; Kwak, 1987; Whong, 1987).

If pregnancy is suspected at any time following sterilization, the woman should be carefully evaluated for evidence of ectopic pregnancy. Sterilization providers must be able to refer clients with suspected ectopic pregnancies to another facility if necessary. Clients and community field-workers should be aware of this condition and should be aware of the need to obtain immediate medical attention if any of the following symptoms occurs (Stewart et al., 1987):

- Sudden intense pain, persistent pain, or cramping in the lower abdomen, usually localized to one side.
- Irregular bleeding or spotting with abdominal pain after a missed or abnormally light menstrual period.
- Fainting or dizziness that persists for more than a few seconds, which could indicate internal bleeding. (Vaginal bleeding does not necessarily accompany internal bleeding associated with ectopic pregnancy.)

Reporting procedures

Female sterilization services should develop a standardized system for reporting and investigating any major complications and deaths that occur. Responsibility for reporting, investigating, and follow-up of these events should be clearly delineated and carefully followed. This system can be a valuable tool in management, in monitoring and supervision of medical services, and in quality assurance activities (see page 160).

13. Effectiveness

Female sterilization is a highly effective method of contraception, and this is undoubtedly important to the increasing numbers of women who are choosing it. Sterilization failures (pregnancies after the procedure) occur in less than 1% of women in the first year after surgery for the most widely used techniques. By comparison, recent studies in the United States have shown that the failure rates associated with many temporary methods of contraception are much higher (see Table 3, page 12).

Failures have been reported with all methods of tubal occlusion up to several years after surgery; however, the majority occur within the first one or two years. Most reported failure rates for postpartum and interval minilaparotomy procedures using the Pomeroy technique are in the range of 0.2–0.4% in the first year (Cheng et al., 1977; Chi et al., 1980; M. Trías, personal communication, 1984). Longer-term follow-up failure rates remain low—0.3% at 24 months (Cheng et al., 1977), although one study reported 0.8% at 36 months (M. Trías, personal communication, 1984). Most failure rates for interval procedures using bands vary from 0.4% to 0.7%, and a few small studies of bands applied postpartum have reported rates in the range of 0.6–1.5% (Bhiwandiwala et al., 1982; Chi et al., 1980, 1981; Mumford & Bhiwandiwala, 1981; M. Trías, personal communication, 1984). Studies of interval laparoscopic procedures using bands have shown failure rates of 0.5% at 24 months (Bhiwandiwala et al., 1982) and 1.3% at 36 months (M. Trías, personal communication, 1984).

However, it is difficult to make valid comparisons between the different techniques. Studies often use different measures of effectiveness and sometimes do not control for such variables as the technical skill and experience of surgeons, the timing of the procedure, the length of time following surgery, and the occlusive technique used. The experience of the surgeon is often a more important determinant of failure rates than inherent differences among techniques.

Reasons for failure

Pregnancy following female sterilization may be the result of conception occurring before the procedure, spontaneous reconnection (recanalization) of the ends of the fallopian tube, or the formation of fistulas (abnormal openings in the tubal wall) after surgery. Surgical errors and technical problems may also lead to some pregnancies. Both the surgical approach and the technique of occlusion can influence the success or failure of the procedure.

Pre-existing pregnancy

During the postovulatory, or luteal, phase of the menstrual cycle, after a fertilized egg has already passed through the tubes of the uterus, a woman may be pregnant even though she has not yet missed her period. Various studies have indicated that such pregnancies, unrecognized at the time of female sterilization, account for between 8% and 45% of all pregnancies reported after sterilization (Liskin et al., 1985).

These pregnancies do not result from sterilization failure, since conception preceded the operation. However, the woman may still perceive that the sterilization has failed, so some service providers try to avoid operating on women at this stage of the menstrual cycle. Close supervision and careful attention to preoperative medical screening, as well as provision of services in the immediate postpartum or postabortion period, will reduce the number of pregnant women undergoing sterilization. Sterilization procedures should also be scheduled for the preovulatory phase of the menstrual cycle wherever possible. The small risk that a woman is already pregnant in the latter half of her cycle must be weighed against the chances that she will become pregnant if the procedure is delayed, or that she may become discouraged and not persist in obtaining her chosen method of contraception if required to wait. If the couple is not using contraception and the medical staff believe or suspect that the woman may be pregnant, a pregnancy test should be performed, if possible (WFHAAVSC, 1988). In any case, the woman should be informed that she may be pregnant before the sterilization, and a record kept of the conversation.

Routine dilatation and curettage or vacuum aspiration immediately prior to sterilization to rule out pregnancy is not recommended. This additional procedure increases both the risk of infection and the time and cost of the sterilization. However, the routine removal of an IUD at the time of sterilization, which does not require the use of antibiotics, is accepted practice.

Spontaneous recanalization and fistula formation

Spontaneous rejoining of the fallopian tubes and fistula formation are rare events leading to pregnancy after sterilization. The causes are not completely known and are difficult to determine unless the condition of the tubes can be observed during a second sterilization or other pelvic operation. The method used to occlude the tubes may affect the incidence of these events. Unipolar electrocoagulation appears to have a higher rate of failure due to fistula formation than other commonly used occlusive methods (Whong, 1987). Proper application of clips and bands, on the correct section of the tube, with adequate tension will prevent most failures related to these occlusive techniques. The use of catgut for ligation in Pomeroy procedures is important to allow the cut ends of the tube to be separated, which reduces the likelihood of recanalization. Some authorities strongly recommend plain catgut (Pritchard et al., 1985), although in practice the more slowly resorbed chromic catgut is widely used with generally satisfactory results.

Surgical errors and technical problems

Up to 30–50% of sterilization failures in a number of studies have been attributed to surgical errors (Liskin et al., 1985). One frequent cause of these failures—occlusion of the incorrect structure (such as the round ligament)—can be avoided by careful identification of the fimbria of each tube before occlusion. Failures may also occur if mechanical occlusive devices are applied to the wrong portion of the tube, if clips are not correctly positioned or locked (across the entire tube), or if the tube is not completely coagulated during electrocoagulation procedures. Inadequate coagulation may be a more common problem with bipolar than with unipolar equipment. Most of these errors occur during or shortly after training, when the surgeon is inexperienced in the technique being used. One study indicated that the first 100 women undergoing sterilization at a centre with recently trained surgeons were three times more likely to become pregnant than women sterilized later (Chi et al., 1980).

Pregnancies may also occur after sterilization if technical problems, such as equipment malfunction, cause clips or bands to be incorrectly applied so that the tube is not fully occluded or the device comes off. Silicone bands may also be torn or cut when being placed on applicators, such that they will not fully occlude the tube or will slip off. Problems with the lens or light source of the laparoscope can contribute to surgical errors where a device is incorrectly applied or placed on the wrong structure.

14. Reversal[1]

Female sterilization should not be offered or promoted as a reversible method of fertility control. While it is feasible to perform reconstructive surgery to reverse sterilization, and several countries have developed the capacity to provide reversal services, the proportion of clients who request a reversal and subsequently achieve a successful pregnancy is quite low.

Reasons and potential demand for reversal requests

While the large majority of clients who elect to undergo sterilization remain satisfied with their choice, a few clients are likely to change their mind and express interest in re-establishing their fertility through reversal surgery. This may be because of unexpected changes in their individual circumstances, such as the death of a child, remarriage, or an improved socioeconomic status. Conceivably, the number of requests for reversal will increase as sterilization becomes increasingly popular, particularly among younger age groups and lower-parity groups, and as people become more aware of the availability of sterilization reversal services.

Since data are not systematically collected and analysed, it is very difficult to obtain reliable estimates of the potential demand for reversal of sterilization. Nevertheless, a recent survey suggests that in developing countries 1–3 individuals per 1000 who have been sterilized will later seek reversal. In developed countries, according to data from Canada and the United States of America, this proportion may be as high as 1–3 per 100 (Marcil-Gratton, 1988; Moss & Association for Voluntary Surgical

[1] Parts of this chapter have been adapted from *Sterilization reversal: issues and implications for voluntary surgical contraception programs*, to be published by the Association for Voluntary Surgical Contraception, forthcoming.

Contraception, 1988). In any case, estimates by providers of reversal services may understate the true level of demand, since in many settings reversal services are not available or clients lack information and knowledge about them.

Service considerations

Reversal surgery involves sophisticated techniques and skills, as well as high costs, and is not guaranteed to be available, appropriate, or successful for those clients who might desire it. Thus, managers must deal with a number of service issues when considering establishing or managing reversal services, which are outlined below.

Success rates

Numerous investigators have reported on the success rates for female sterilization reversal. Many have found encouragingly high success rates (see Association for Voluntary Surgical Contraception, forthcoming, and Liskin et al., 1985, for summaries and discussions of these studies). However, these reported high success rates can be misleading if not carefully analysed.

From the perspectives of the provider and of the client who wishes to have her fertility restored, the goal of reversal should be to achieve an intrauterine pregnancy resulting in the delivery of a live baby. However, success in achieving this goal is often not what is assessed and reported in the literature. Instead, many researchers have defined "success" as the achievement of tubal patency or pregnancy, regardless of the outcome. Furthermore, some studies do not include women who request reversal but are rejected because, among other reasons, they are considered unsuitable candidates, fail to meet service selection criteria, or cannot afford the costs.

As a result, reported success rates may give misleading encouragement to individuals interested in reversal. Fig. 9 illustrates why many clients requesting reversal may never experience a successful outcome as indicated by an intrauterine pregnancy that results in the delivery of a live baby. Therefore, service providers should not quote or advertise success rates, since these rates may have little relevance to a particular client's chance of a successful reversal.

Fig. 9. Scheme for assessing the outcome of requests for female sterilization reversal surgery

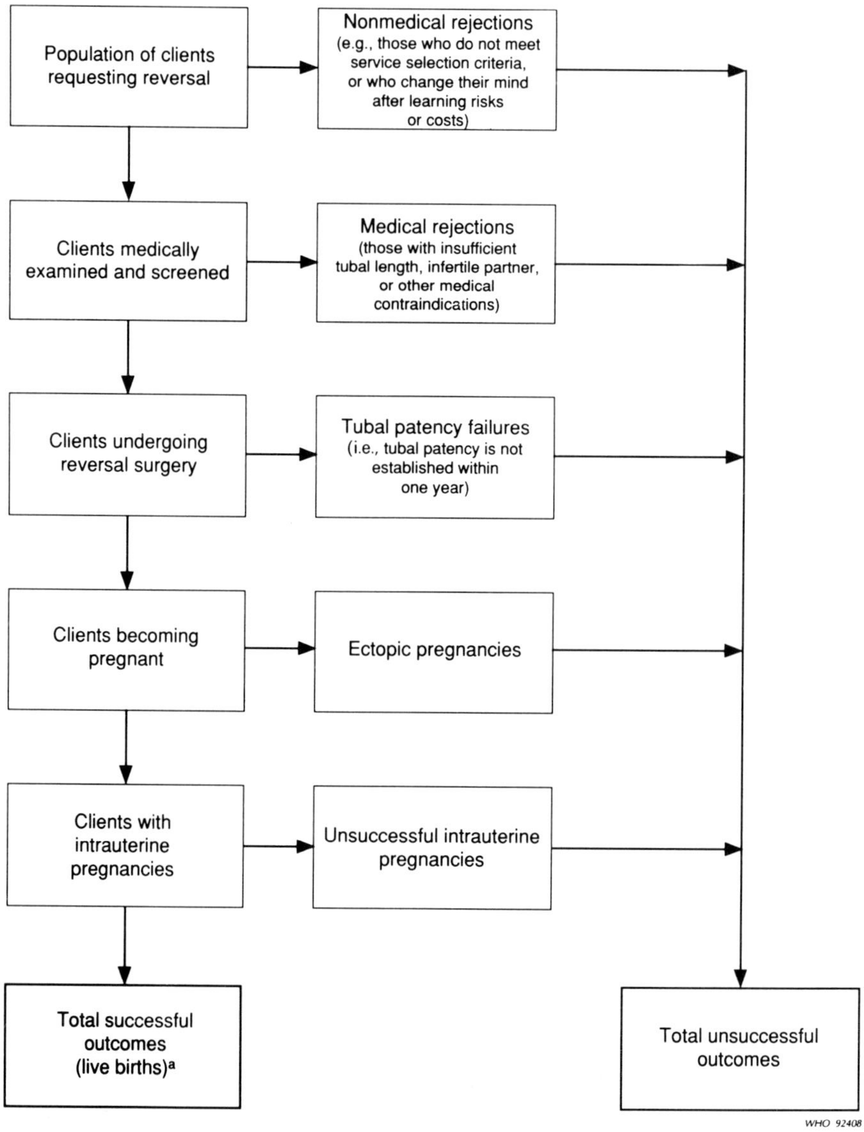

[a] From a clinical perspective, reversal surgery is successful when intrauterine pregnancies are achieved, since the inability to carry a pregnancy to term is not caused by the reversal procedure. However, from the client's perspective, success would generally be associated with a live birth.

Factors influencing the success of reversal

Reversal surgery is more likely to be successful if an occlusive technique that minimized the degree of damage to the tubes was used when the sterilization surgery was performed (see Table 16). For example, clips usually destroy the smallest amount of tube and are associated with the highest proportion of intrauterine pregnancies (89%) following reversal. Rates of pregnancy following reversal surgery decline successively with the use of bands, Pomeroy technique, electrocoagulation, Irving technique, and fimbriectomy. However, these rates should be interpreted with caution, as explained earlier. In any case, if reversal services are made available, providers will need to consider carefully which techniques of tubal occlusion should be promoted as the standard techniques. Although clips may offer the best chance for successful reversal, they are also more expensive than bands and ligation.

Successful reversal may also depend on the site of occlusion. Studies suggest that isthmic-isthmic and cornual-isthmic anastomoses increase the chances of success. With cornual-isthmic anastomosis, a larger portion of distal tube remains intact. Isthmic-isthmic anastomosis is, however, easier to perform, because the portions being anastomosed are of similar diameter. Furthermore, ampullary anastomosis appears to be

Table 16. Intrauterine pregnancy rate following reversal surgery

Occlusive technique	No. of studies	No. of women in studies[a]	Intrauterine pregnancy rate (%)[b]	Range of rates (%)
Clips (spring, Filshie)	11	188	89	50–100
Silicone bands	14	251	74	50–100
Pomeroy ligation	16	712	63	35–74
Electrocoagulation (unipolar and bipolar)	17	653	55	21–83
Irving ligation	6	29	48	33–75
Fimbriectomy	5	30	27	0–44

[a] These studies do not include women who request reversal but are rejected for medical or service-related reasons, are unable to afford the costs, or decide not to go ahead with the reversal, for whatever reason.

[b] Includes pregnancies that did not result in term deliveries.

Source: Adapted from Association for Voluntary Surgical Contraception, forthcoming.

associated with a higher proportion of ectopic pregnancies (Hulka & Halme, 1988; Rock et al., 1982; Spivak et al., 1986).

Reversal surgery has become more successful with the introduction of microsurgical techniques, which minimize the degree of tissue trauma and facilitate accurate dissection, realignment, and suturing. The procedure is usually performed under general anaesthesia.[1]

Cost considerations

The cost to family planning services of providing reversal services is high, particularly in relation to the number of clients who are likely to benefit from them. A significant initial investment may be needed to train reversal specialists, procure microsurgery equipment and instruments, and set up an animal laboratory where the surgeons can practise and maintain their skills. In addition, substantial recurring expenses must be met, including those for the maintenance of animal laboratories and microsurgery equipment, the replenishment of expendable supplies, especially very fine suture material, which is expensive, and basic operational costs, such as personnel salaries and operating theatre time.

Other health policy issues related to costs must also be considered. If resources for basic health services are scarce, planners and managers must weigh the costs of establishing and maintaining reversal services for a small number of clients against investments in other important health needs, such as expanding primary health care and family planning services, which will benefit considerably more people. Furthermore, to maintain their skills, surgeons require continuing practice and operating time that must be obtained at the expense of other reproductive health services. Service providers must consider how best to use the time of a limited number of specialists and how best to allocate scarce operating theatre time.

From the economic perspective of society and of clients, the number of reversal services should be kept to a minimum. Thorough preoperative counselling of clients is therefore essential to identify those most likely to change their mind after surgery. Such clients require additional counselling and providers may

---

[1] For further details see Henry et al., 1980; Hunt, 1986; Phillips, 1981; and Sciarra et al., 1978.

need to deny them sterilization services and inform them about temporary methods of contraception (see pages 61 and 73).

Location of services

In general, reversal services should be restricted to major surgical centres to ensure that the surgeons have the volume of cases, the trained assistants, and the equipment necessary to maintain high-quality services. Systems for referring clients to these centres should also be developed to meet the demand for reversal in rural areas (Association for Voluntary Surgical Contraception, forthcoming).

Family planning services must also decide whether, and to what extent, clients should pay for reversal surgery. If clients are asked to contribute a large proportion of the costs, it is likely that fewer women will be able to afford the procedure.

Counselling and reversal services

In countries where reversal services are not widely available or well known to the general public, the subject of sterilization reversal need be discussed only if a client considering sterilization raises the question or expresses an interest in reversal. Where reversal services are well established, or where reversal is widely believed to be available, all potential sterilization clients should receive accurate information about it during counselling. This information should also be given to clients who express an interest in reversal after sterilization. Counselling about reversal should cover the following points:

- Reversal surgery is expensive, difficult, time-consuming, usually involves the use of general anaesthesia, and is not guaranteed to result in subsequent pregnancy.
- Following surgery, the client can expect to experience more pain or discomfort and will require a longer period of recovery than after sterilization.
- Reversal surgery poses more risks to the client than sterilization.
- Many clients who request reversal are rejected because of their age, fertility impairments, their partner's age or infertility, damage to or insufficient length of fallopian tube, or contraindications to pregnancy.

- The risk of ectopic pregnancy, which is life-threatening, is higher than average after reversal surgery.

Potential clients for sterilization who remain interested in reversal after counselling are not suitable candidates for sterilization.

Client screening

Client screening is an integral component of reversal services. In addition to counselling (as described above), the screening process for the woman should include a medical history, a physical examination including laparoscopy, a test for ovulation, appropriate laboratory tests, and a review of the sterilization operative report (if available). The fertility of her partner should also be assessed. Since fertility declines with age, the age of both the client and her partner must be considered. Some reversal services do not accept clients who are over 37 years of age.

Most reversal surgeons consider laparoscopy to be mandatory before reversal surgery. This procedure enables the surgeon to determine the condition of the fallopian tubes and fimbriae, whether the woman has any pelvic adhesions that might interfere with reversal surgery, and whether sufficient tube is available to allow reversal. At least 4 cm of the distal portion of the tube should be available if a reversal is to be attempted.

Alternatives to reversal

Clients who are not suitable candidates for reversal may wish to investigate other options, such as adoption or *in vitro* fertilization. However, these are not normally feasible, can be very expensive, and may not be available. Thus, further counselling of couples who wish to pursue these options may be required to ensure that they are emotionally and financially prepared to undergo the difficulties they will almost certainly encounter. Couples who continue to express a strong desire for children and who wish to pursue *in vitro* fertilization should understand that this technique is associated with a low rate of success and is usually more expensive than reversal surgery. Adoption may be a more realistic alternative if it is culturally acceptable and if procedures and institutions to arrange it are in place.

15. The setting

The setting or physical facility for female sterilization services should be designed and managed to achieve three objectives—to permit delivery of high-quality medical services; to be responsive to client needs, thus leading to a high level of comfort and satisfaction; and to provide services efficiently and cost-effectively.

Service facilities

Female sterilization can be offered in a variety of permanent and temporary locations, as discussed in Chapter 3. However, regardless of where female sterilizations are performed, the facility should include the following:

- a reception and registration area,
- a comfortable waiting area for clients,
- space for counselling that allows for privacy,
- an examination room, for preoperative and follow-up examinations, including changing facilities for clients,
- restricted areas where surgical personnel can change clothes and scrub before surgery,
- a comfortable, private waiting area for clients before surgery,
- a sterile room for surgery, isolated from the outside and from clinic traffic,
- toilet and washing facilities for clients and staff (preferably separate facilities),
- a recovery area for clients after surgery,
- facilities for cleaning, sterilizing, and autoclaving surgical instruments, equipment, linen, and dressings,

- space for storage of records, supplies, and equipment,
- arrangements for laboratory investigations,
- a laundry.

Often one area is used for several purposes, but the facility must have sufficient space for each activity, arranged so as to allow for efficient client flow (see page 134). Some of the activities listed above, such as laboratory tests, laundry, and autoclaving, may be contracted out or, in multipurpose services, handled by a central supply unit.

Good lighting, electricity, and a clean water supply are desirable for the provision of high-quality sterilization services. However, in rural and remote locations, it is possible to perform minilaparotomy without a permanent source of electricity. In these situations, a generator or electric torches should be available. A reliable source of electricity is indispensable for laparoscopy services. While it is preferable to have clean tap-water for washing, scrub-up procedures, cleaning instruments, and sanitation, services may use alternative clean water supplies if necessary.

Clients should not be allowed to move freely through the service facility. To promote proper cleanliness, infection control, and efficiency, the facility should be divided into three areas, as described below and summarized in Table 17.

Table 17. Space allocation for various functions and activities in a female sterilization service, according to degree of restriction

Unrestricted area	Semi-restricted area	Restricted area
Reception Registration Information Counselling Waiting area Storage of records and non-sterile equipment and supplies Public toilet	Laboratory tests Sterilization of equipment and supplies Storage of sterile equipment and supplies Toilet and changing facilities for staff and clients Examination rooms (preoperative and follow-up) Preoperative waiting area Recovery area	Scrub area Operating theatre Other sterile procedures

Unrestricted area

Street clothes are permitted in this general area. Activities carried out here are reception and registration of clients, and information and counselling procedures. This area should also be used for storing records and non-sterile equipment and supplies. A waiting area and toilet facilities for clients should be located here as well.

Semi-restricted area

Any staff entering the semi-restricted area should wear uniforms, laboratory coats, or scrub attire. Equipment and supplies should be sterilized in this area, which is also used for storing clean and sterile supplies and instruments. This area should also incorporate toilet and changing facilities for staff and clients having surgery, facilities for performing laboratory tests, examination rooms, preoperative waiting rooms, and post-operative recovery areas.

After surgery, it should be possible for clients to reach the recovery area without passing through the preoperative waiting area. The recovery area must be sufficiently large to accommodate all clients who may be recovering at any one time and to allow staff to move freely to monitor their vital signs.

Restricted area

This area should be considered an isolation zone, which may be entered only by staff wearing scrub attire. This area includes the scrub area, the operating theatre, and areas where other sterile procedures are carried out. Only essential movement into and out of the area should be allowed, especially when surgery is in progress. A barrier or clearly marked buffer zone may be used to discourage traffic between contaminated areas of the facility and this restricted area; however, the area should be readily accessible in case of emergency. The operating theatre should be kept locked when not in use and should not be used as a general storage area.

If a service-delivery facility is to be constructed or renovated, it may be useful to include a doctor in the planning team to ensure that the required space is allocated and designed appropriately.

Client flow

An orderly flow of clients through the female sterilization service facility is essential to ensure a comprehensive, cost-effective service and to enhance client satisfaction. An efficient system for attending to clients also contributes to proper infection control and maintenance of facilities; this becomes even more critical as the case-load increases.

A diagram depicting the typical flow of clients at a service site is given in Fig. 10. The scheduling and movement of clients through the service facility should be organized as efficiently as possible to minimize the waiting time for clients and to make the best use of staff time. Factors to be considered in planning client flow include the duration of each clinic session, the services

Fig. 10. Typical client flow in a female sterilization service

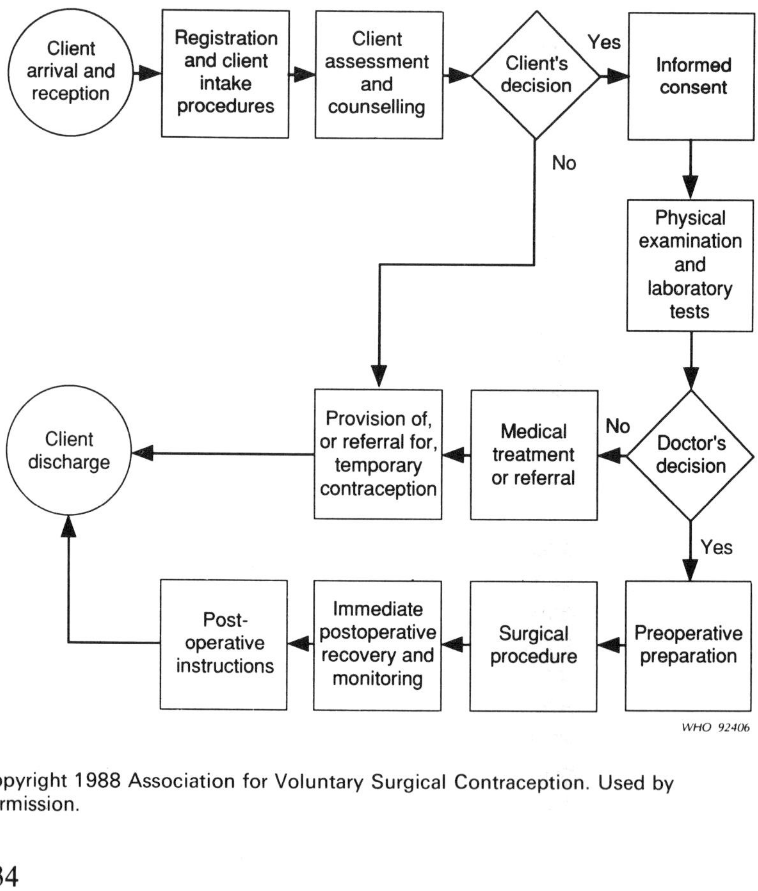

provided during each session, the availability and number of staff, the number of clients scheduled or expected per session, and the physical design of the clinic. In many countries, service managers have used a technique developed by the Centers for Disease Control in the United States of America, known as patient-flow analysis, to identify problems and bottlenecks in clinic scheduling procedures and in the physical layout of the facility (see Edmunds et al., 1987).

The scheme outlined in Fig. 10 may differ slightly for postpartum and postabortion services, in that some of the procedures may have taken place before admission for delivery or pregnancy termination. It is important to note that a certain number of clients entering the service site for sterilization may be rejected on medical or other grounds, or may decide against the procedure after receiving additional information and counselling. Consequently, service staff must be able to provide alternative methods of contraception and medical treatment for these women or to refer them elsewhere for these services. Arrangements must also be made for clients who return for follow-up or for resupply of temporary contraceptives.

Prevention of infection

Infection control is governed in part by the appropriate allocation and segregation of space in the service facility (see Table 18). However, the incidence of serious infection can be significantly reduced if guidelines outlining appropriate and effective aseptic routines are established and closely followed. Adherence to the guidelines should be closely monitored by supervisors.

The operating theatre

In stationary clinics, the operating theatre should have a tile or concrete floor that can be easily and thoroughly cleaned. The room should be enclosed to keep it free of dust and flying insects, and air-conditioned if possible. Air-conditioners should be placed high, and the airflow should be directed away from the surgical field. In the absence of air-conditioning, ceiling or floor fans may be used if absolutely necessary; these should also be positioned to ensure that the airflow is directed away from the surgical field. If fans are used, they must be cleaned regularly.

Table 18. Recommended methods of sterilization and disinfection of instruments and supplies

Materials[a]	Method	
Linens	Steam sterilization	1 atmosphere (101 kPa, 15 lb/in^2) above atmospheric pressure, 121 °C (250 °F) for 30 min
Rubber goods[b]	Steam sterilization	1 atmosphere (101 kPa, 15 lb/in^2) above atmospheric pressure, 121 °C (250 °F) for 15–20 min
	Immersion in chemical disinfectant	Immersion in glutaral (glutaraldehyde) 2% aqueous alkaline solution for 10 hours (for sterilization) or 30 min (for high-level disinfection)
Surgical instruments[b]	Steam sterilization	1 atmosphere (101 kPa, 15 lb/in^2) above atmospheric pressure, 121 °C (250 °F) for 30 min
	Dry heat sterilization	170 °C (340 °F) for 120 min
	Immersion in chemical disinfectant[c]	Immersion in glutaral (glutaraldehyde) 2% aqueous alkaline solution for 10 hours (for sterilization) or 30 min (for high-level disinfection)
	Boiling (for high-level disinfection)	Boiling for 20 min in a closed container

[a] Unwrapped sterile surgical instruments and other supplies should be used immediately. If wrapped, they should remain sterile for up to one week.

[b] Following surgery, all surgical instruments and reusable gloves should be immediately immersed in an appropriate low-level or intermediate chemical disinfectant (e.g. sodium hypochlorite solution, 5% available chlorine) for 10 minutes to remove traces of blood and body fluids.

[c] This method must not be used for needles and syringes, and should only be used for other skin-cutting and invasive instruments if neither sterilization nor high-level disinfection by boiling is possible (see opposite).

Sources: WFHAAVSC, 1988, and WHO, 1989b.

Natural ventilation may also be established through screened windows; these should be at least 1.8 m above the floor.

For temporary and mobile services, the room used for surgery should be selected and located to allow for the maintenance of strict asepsis. The features mentioned above for stationary clinics are also desirable for temporary service facility operating theatres.

Ideally, no operations involving dirty or infected cases should be performed in the same room as female sterilization procedures. If this is unavoidable, the room should be disinfected following surgery on dirty or infected cases. Otherwise, all operating theatres should be scrubbed and disinfected at least once a week on days when no operations are scheduled. If insect infestation is observed, the room should be fumigated.

Sterilization and disinfection of equipment[1]

Sterilization involves the inactivation of all microorganisms, including spores. Disinfection, on the other hand, does not destroy spores. For female sterilization surgery, all equipment must be thoroughly cleaned before it is sterilized or disinfected, using a brush and soapy water, in order to remove any blood and other organic matter that may harbour microorganisms. All linen and equipment, except endoscopic equipment (laparoscopes), should be sterilized in a steam autoclave. If an autoclave is not available, instruments should be sterilized by dry heat. Boiling for 20–30 minutes in a closed container may be used for high-level disinfection of instruments, but is insufficient for the purposes of sterilization. High-level disinfection by immersion in chemical disinfectants must not be used for needles and syringes. Chemical high-level disinfection for other skin-cutting and invasive instruments should only be employed as the last resort if neither sterilization nor high-level disinfection by boiling is possible, and then only if the appropriate concentration and activity of the chemical can be ensured and if the instruments have been thoroughly cleaned prior to immersion. Recommended sterilization and disinfection methods and solutions are presented in Table 18.

Endoscopic equipment is sensitive to heat and should be sterilized by immersion in glutaral (glutaraldehyde) 2% aqueous alkaline solution for 10 hours. Endoscopic instruments should be disassembled, cleaned, and sterilized after each operating session and after every infected case. Between cases, these instruments must receive high-level disinfection by immersion in glutaral

---

[1] For additional information on methods of disinfection and sterilization of instruments and supplies, see Angle, 1989; Porter, 1987; Tietjen & McIntosh, 1989; WFHAAVSC, 1988; and WHO, 1989b. For a comprehensive discussion of the recommended procedures of sterilizing endoscopes, see Altobelli et al., 1980a and 1980b.

(glutaraldehyde) 2% aqueous alkaline solution for 30 minutes. After immersion, all equipment should be thoroughly rinsed with sterile water.

Ethylene oxide gas is effective for sterilizing endoscopic equipment; however, it is expensive and is not available in most settings. Ultraviolet light is not an effective sterilizing agent for this equipment and is not recommended (WFHAAVSC, 1988).

16. Instruments, equipment, and supplies

Appropriate and adequate instruments, equipment, and supplies are crucial for the successful implementation of female sterilization services. A service manager who is concerned with cost-effectiveness as well as medical quality must carefully consider both the necessary capital investment in equipment and instruments and the recurring costs of expendable supplies. In consultation with the medical staff, the manager must determine what equipment, instruments, and supplies will be adequate and appropriate to the setting in which the service is to be delivered and for the techniques of sterilization to be used.

Equipment

Table 19 and Annexes 3 and 4 list the equipment and instruments required to set up a female sterilization service; these items represent capital expenditures. Table 19 is presented according to the various stages of the service: preoperative and follow-up examinations, preoperative preparation, surgery, and recovery.

Examinations

The examination room used for preoperative and follow-up examinations must be equipped with the following: an examination table (with or without knee rests or stirrups), an examination lamp, a stool, and a weighing scale. A cabinet for storing commonly used items may be useful. A haemoglobinometer or centrifuge will be required if tests to measure the erythrocyte volume fraction (haematocrit) are to be performed at the service site. Other items required for this setting include a stethoscope, sphygmomanometer, thermometer, dressing jar, and instruments for conducting basic pelvic examinations, and for removing sutures.

Table 19. Equipment and instruments for female sterilization

	Equipment	Instruments
Preoperative and follow-up examinations	Examination table Examination lamp Stool Weighing scales Dressing jar Storage cabinet[a] Haemoglobinometer or centrifuge[a]	Stethoscope Sphygmomanometer Thermometer Instruments for carrying out pelvic examinations and for removing sutures
Preoperative preparation		
Sterilization and disinfection of instruments and equipment	Autoclave Autoclave drums or containers Instrument pan with cover Dry-heat sterilizer[b] Water boiler[b]	None required
Scrub procedures	Antiseptic-solution dispenser Hand brushes Elbow tap connection[a]	None required
Preparation of client	Stainless steel bowl	Sponge forceps Razor, clippers, or scissors[a]
Surgery	Operating table Operating light Instrument tray Stand for intravenous fluids Waste bucket Small stainless steel bowl Dressing jar Instrument table[a] Instrument cabinet[a] Stool[a] Anaesthesia machine (*or* equipment for intravenous general anaesthesia)[e]	Stethoscope Sphygmomanometer Surgical instruments for specific sterilization approach and technique (see page 142)[c,d]
Recovery	Stretcher or wheelchair[a] Beds or cots with mattresses	Stethoscope Sphygmomanometer Thermometer

[a] Optional equipment.

[b] For use with instruments only; not suitable for linen.

[c] Minilaparotomy surgical instruments are listed in Annex 3. Components of laparoscopy systems are listed in Annex 4.

[d] These items must be sterile.

[e] For services using general anaesthesia either as the principal anaesthetic or as a back-up for local anaesthesia in difficult or complicated cases.

Preoperative preparation

The equipment and supplies required to sterilize or disinfect linen, instruments, and other items used during surgery depend upon the methods of sterilization and disinfection that are chosen. Methods of sterilization and disinfection for various materials are discussed on page 137 and in Table 20.

An antiseptic-solution dispenser and hand brushes are required for the surgical scrub area. Ideally, connectors should be placed on taps so that they can be turned off using the elbow. A stainless steel bowl and sponge forceps are required to prepare clients for surgery. A razor, clippers, or scissors are also required if local practice includes shaving or clipping the operative site.

Operating theatre

All operating theatres that are used for female sterilization should be equipped with an operating table that is adjustable to the head-down (Trendelenburg) position. Many surgeons prefer to use an operating table with a drop end and lithotomy leg supports; however, a drop end is not needed for postpartum cases.

Good lighting is essential for efficient and safe surgery, and the operating light selected for female sterilization procedures must be bright and sharply focused. However, if most procedures will be performed under local anaesthesia, low-intensity ambient lighting assists in relaxing the client.

An instrument tray, stand for intravenous fluids, waste bucket, stethoscope, sphygmomanometer, stainless steel bowl, dressing jar, and syringes are also required for the operating theatre. Items of equipment for use in the operating theatre are listed in Table 19.

Recovery

In services that routinely use local anaesthesia with light sedation, clients are usually able to walk, with assistance, from the operating theatre to the recovery area. In these situations, a hand-carried stretcher or wheelchair should be available for use in emergencies. If general or regional anaesthesia is used, however, a stretcher on wheels will be required. Adequate numbers of simple recovery beds or cots with mattresses are also required. A sphygmomanometer, stethoscope, and thermometer must also be available in this area.

Surgical instruments and endoscopic equipment

The instruments and equipment that are required vary, according to the method of female sterilization used. Instruments and equipment used for minilaparotomy and laparoscopy procedures are discussed below.

Minilaparotomy

Various donor agencies have assembled instrument kits for minilaparotomy, which are available to selected sterilization services. UNICEF, for example, provides a kit which is available to other United Nations agencies and to governmental and recognized nongovernmental agencies. The contents of the minilaparotomy kit provided by UNICEF are listed in Annex 3. The kits can be obtained from UNICEF, UNICEF Plads, Freeport, DK-2100, Copenhagen, Denmark.

Other groups located in developing countries should contact the UNICEF office responsible for services in their respective countries.

The United States Agency for International Development (USAID) also provides kits which are available to both governmental and nongovernmental services. These kits may be obtained through USAID and some of the agencies listed in Annex 1, including the Association for Voluntary Surgical Contraception (AVSC), the JHPIEGO Corporation, and the Pathfinder Fund.

Each clinic should have enough instruments on hand for a typical day's case-load without interruption of the surgical schedule. When determining the number of sets of instruments needed, service managers should consider the time required to resterilize instruments and to allow them to cool to a comfortable temperature. In clinics performing only one or two procedures per operating session, at least two sets should be available. In busier clinics, with case-loads of five to ten operations per day, up to ten sets are recommended so that staff members do not need to resterilize instruments until the end of the day. However, where case-loads exceed ten operations per day, it may be impractical and too expensive to have one set of instruments for every procedure performed. In these cases, it is suggested that one set of minilaparotomy instruments should be available for every two procedures, and that arrangements should be made to sterilize the instruments after each operation.

Laparoscopy

The specific equipment required to carry out female sterilization using laparoscopy is determined by the type of laparoscopic procedure performed (see page 14), the laparoscopic technique employed by the surgeon (single- or double-puncture), the method of tubal occlusion (e.g., bands, clips, or electrocoagulation), and whether the equipment will be used solely for sterilization purposes or also for diagnosis and other surgical procedures. Annex 4 lists the instruments and equipment that are needed to perform a typical laparoscopy procedure, together with a source of addresses of several suppliers of endoscopic equipment.

In case of an emergency, laparoscopy services must have the facilities and properly trained staff to administer general anaesthesia. Anaesthetic apparatus must be available in the operating theatre, unless general anaesthesia is to be administered via intravenous drugs (e.g., ketamine). A full set of laparotomy instruments should be available, sterilized, and ready to use in all laparoscopy services in case an endoscopic procedure must be abandoned and completed by means of laparotomy. The UNICEF and the USAID minilaparotomy kits, with the addition of one set of large retractors, are appropriate for performing laparotomy. If electrocoagulation is to be used, a special electrosurgical unit is required. However, this technique is not recommended as a standard occlusive technique.

Supplies

Table 20 lists all the supplies needed for female sterilization services. These items are listed according to whether they are needed preoperatively, postoperatively, or during surgery.

The quantity of supplies required is determined by the total number of clients and the daily case-load (see page 36 for methods of calculating the potential case-load). For example, supplies that are sterilized between procedures (such as syringes, needles, surgical blades, non-disposable gloves, and linen) must be purchased in adequate quantities to allow the surgical schedule to be completed without interruption. These items should also be stocked in adequate quantities so that any items that are broken or worn out can be replaced immediately.

Disposable or consumable items such as drugs, disposable gloves, suture materials, antiseptic solutions, and gauze must also

Table 20. Supplies for female sterilization[a]

	Supplies
Preoperative and follow-up examinations	Gloves (disposable or non-disposable) Glove powder Table covers Sponges or swabs Materials for laboratory tests (if performed at service site)
Preoperative preparation	
Sterilization and disinfection of instruments	Detergent Disinfectant Sterilizing solution
Scrub procedures	Soap Antiseptic solution
Preparation of client	Razor blades[b] Sponges or swabs Soap Antiseptic solution
Surgery	Gloves (non-disposable)[c] Glove powder Surgical caps, gowns, and masks[c] Surgical drapes[c] Table covers[c] Gauze[c] Adhesive tape Intravenous fluids and administration sets with large-calibre needles[c] Needles for local anaesthesia[c] Surgical blades[c] Suture needles and material[c] Sponges or swabs[c] Silicone bands or clips[b,c]

[a] Drugs required for anaesthesia and emergencies are noted in Chapter 9.
[b] This item is optional.
[c] This item must be sterile.

be purchased in adequate quantities to cover service needs for several weeks, if possible. One pair of clips or silicone bands will be required for each case, if these methods of occlusion are used; extra clips or bands should be on hand in the event of breakage.

Emergency equipment

The resuscitation and emergency equipment outlined below must be in good working order, sterilized as required, and readily available for use. This equipment must be accessible to both the operating theatre and the recovery area.

- Manual resuscitator with face mask
- Oxygen cylinder with a suitable pressure-reducing valve, flow meter, rubber tubing, and face mask
- Suction apparatus (manual) with tubing and two traps
- Nasopharyngeal airways (two sizes)
- Oropharyngeal airways (two sizes)
- Intravenous fluids and sterile administration sets with large-calibre needles
- Emergency drugs[a]
- A full set of sterilized laparotomy instruments
- Anaesthetic apparatus or intravenous anaesthetic drugs (e.g., ketamine)—recommended for minilaparotomy training programmes and laparoscopy services

[a] These include naloxone, epinephrine, diphenhydramine, atropine, diazepam, lidocaine, sodium bicarbonate solution, physostigmine, and flumazenil. This list may be extended or modified on the basis of the anaesthesia used and local medical practices.

If staff have been trained in intubation and the use of a laryngoscope, a laryngoscope and a full set of endotracheal tubes should also be available. Otherwise, oral or nasopharyngeal airways and manual resuscitators with face masks should be used for resuscitation (see page 96).

Other equipment and materials

Other equipment, furnishings, and supplies required by female sterilization services include items such as benches, chairs, tables, and desks for the reception and waiting areas, as well as filing cabinets and other furniture for storing service records, charts, supplies, and equipment. In addition, client information materials (see pages 49–54), informed-consent forms, stationery, and cleaning supplies will be needed.

Maintenance and logistics

The amounts of drugs, suture material, and other expendables required for each case will be established with experience and careful monitoring of the service. However, until experience allows a more site-specific calculation, managers should estimate these requirements in consultation with the surgical staff.

When ordering equipment and supplies, managers must allow adequate time to acquire and install the items. Services should consider obtaining items locally if possible, since imported goods are often slow to arrive and they also tend to be more expensive than local products.

Service managers are responsible for ensuring compliance with any instructions for storing and maintaining equipment and supplies. Training is required in order to maintain laparoscopic equipment, and staff should also know where to go if the equipment needs to be repaired.

Service staff must pay close attention to drug expiry dates and proper storage conditions for drugs and other supplies that are sensitive to temperature and humidity, including pills, condoms, and other methods of temporary contraception. The inventory of expendable supplies must be monitored regularly to ensure that services are not hampered by disruptions in the supply line.

17. Training[1]

A high-quality female sterilization service depends upon well-trained personnel: doctors, surgical assistants and theatre attendants (usually nurses or midwives), counsellors, clinic- and community-based educators, and clinic managers. Sometimes one individual may perform more than one of these roles, such as when a nurse who assists the surgeon also acts as the counsellor or clinic manager.

In any case, all personnel must acquire the knowledge and competence needed to perform the duties assigned to them. Service managers should therefore ensure that training programmes are organized and function to provide appropriate training to each of the above categories.

In addition to ensuring that personnel have the skills required to deliver services, training should produce in the trainees an understanding of, concern for, and commitment to the provision of high-quality services. Accordingly, standards will need to be established for training programmes, since trainees will learn from the example provided by training centres with regard to dealing with clients, organizing services, counselling, and surgical and clinical practices, and will apply what they have learned to their local service sites.

When properly designed and situated, a training programme for sterilization services can serve as the stimulus for further development and improvements in service standards and delivery systems. This happens when training programmes receive feedback relating to the performance of past trainees through a process of data collection, supervision and monitoring, and on-site follow-up. In general, supervision, monitoring, and evaluation activities should be closely linked with training, since

---

[1] For further information about surgical training in sterilization, see *Training guidelines for voluntary surgical contraception*, 1986, and *Safe and voluntary surgical contraception*, 1988, both published by the World Federation of Health Agencies for the Advancement of Voluntary Surgical Contraception.

any problems detected can often be dealt with in initial, refresher, and in-service training courses.

Developing training programmes

There is a continual need for skilled and knowledgeable personnel. While training is an obvious prerequisite when services are being introduced, it is no less important in well-established services, which must periodically replace personnel, conduct refresher and in-service training, upgrade skills, and introduce technological improvements and new standards. Service managers should therefore give priority to the development of appropriate training programmes.

Whether for new or for well-established services, high-quality training must incorporate certain features, including:

- staff who are experienced and competent in female sterilization training;
- knowledge- and skills-based curricula;
- an adequate case-load for each trainee to observe and practise his or her skills, especially for staff being trained in surgery or counselling;
- adequate equipment, materials, and other training resources;
- an appropriate setting.

In many countries, these requirements may be difficult to meet when services are being introduced and temporary measures are frequently needed. For example, if training facilities are not available, the first few service-delivery teams of doctors, surgical assistants, and counsellors may need to be trained in another country, where services are well established and the minimum training requirements can be met. Ideally, some of these personnel will eventually become trainers in their own countries and will establish the first training courses. The curricula for these initial training courses may be adapted from established curricula of other countries, or from international guidelines (see page 157).

Another problem often encountered by new services is that of ensuring an adequate case-load for staff being trained in surgery and counselling. Each trainee should be given adequate opportunity to observe experienced staff members and to practise his or her skills. However, this may not be possible, particularly when services are being introduced, and various adjustments or compensations may be required. For example, the number of trainees may need to be kept low and the training period itself extended. Appointments for clients may need to be scheduled to coincide with training courses. Sometimes client referrals from other sites can also be arranged to compensate for an inadequate case-load at the training site. Some training programmes provide theoretical training to groups of trainees, and practical training for one trainee at a time over several weeks or even months. These measures require extra effort and close attention to detail in order to be successful, and should be regarded as temporary solutions and a means of progressing towards the long-range goal of achieving a sufficiently high and constant case-load at the training site itself.

The location, or institutional base, of the training centres for female sterilization must also be considered. Training programmes have been located in a variety of settings, including medical, nursing, and midwifery schools, university teaching hospitals, specialized governmental training centres, and nongovernmental service organizations, such as national family planning associations. Some countries require that all training and certification activities take place at a single designated training centre, while others permit or encourage the different service-delivery sectors (e.g., governmental, nongovernmental, private, or missionary) to establish individual training programmes and centres. Further, depending on individual country circumstances, training programmes may be geographically centralized or decentralized.

Regardless of the location and design of the training programme that eventually evolves, a long-range concern that must be addressed is how high-quality training can be sustained, or institutionalized, so that training courses are available to fill gaps in personnel requirements whenever needed. Eventually national training standards must be established (see page 150). While donor agencies may offer funds and technical assistance to establish training programmes, these agencies are not usually able to cover the costs of training in the long term. Ideally governments should include the costs of female sterilization training in their annual budgets.

To make essential training more affordable, it may be integrated into existing health services, ideally maternal and child health/family planning services. For example, some countries have located training programmes for female sterilization in university teaching hospitals or medical schools where teaching staff, space, and other resources are already available. However, in such institutions, personnel are often already busy with other teaching responsibilities, and the case-load may not be adequate for training unless the facility has a dedicated family planning clinic and service programme.

There is no uniform prescription for establishing national training programmes for sterilization services. Innovative responses are required according to the particular circumstances, characteristics, and problems of each country.

Training curricula

Knowledge, skills, and specific topics that need to be addressed during sterilization training programmes include the following:

- family planning,
- free and informed choice,
- community information and outreach services,
- clinical support activities,
- medical and surgical procedures,
- management.

A more detailed definition of these topics is given in Table 21. The table also indicates which personnel need to be trained in each specific topic. The table can be used as a basis for developing curricula for the theoretical and practical training for each category of personnel.

Assuring the quality of training

Client satisfaction

All personnel involved in delivering services should regard client satisfaction as a main objective. Training programmes should stress the importance of this ethic, and should reinforce the message by setting an example in the ways in which they are organized and conducted.

The practical training components for doctors, surgical assistants, and counsellors involve dealing with clients. All training activities involving clients must be designed to ensure that:

- Services are well organized, as indicated by accessibility, an orderly flow of clients, and availability of adequate staff and supplies.
- Staff show respect towards clients.
- Personnel are familiar with and sensitive to local culture and customs.
- Staff offer clients reassurance and understanding.

Because of the additional demands and stress placed on staff working at clinical service sites during training programmes, the above features may be compromised. Trainers and managers of clinics where training takes place must remain sensitive to these issues and ensure that trainees are well supervised in their interactions with and treatment of clients. Furthermore, clients should be informed that their procedure will take place in the context of training, and if they do not wish to be treated by trainees, their wishes should be respected (Edmunds et al., 1987).

Requirements for trainers

Knowledge about and skills in the subjects they teach are, of course, prerequisites for trainers. In general, trainers must be qualified in their respective subjects, and they must practise their skills regularly. For example, trainers in laparoscopy must be qualified obstetrician-gynaecologists or general surgeons; trainers in minilaparotomy must be qualified medical practitioners with extensive experience in performing the procedure and should perform at least 10 procedures per month (WFHAAVSC, 1986). Likewise, trainers of counsellors should be experienced in counselling and in training.

Regardless of the subject being taught, all staff providing instruction should have a suitable temperament for training and have the knowledge and skills to train adults using the most effective methods available.

Criteria for selecting trainees

Every training programme should establish and enforce minimum entry requirements for training programmes. Different criteria will need to be set for the various categories of personnel

Table 21. Content of training programmes for personnel in female sterilization services[a]

Knowledge, skills, and specific topics	Surgeon	Clinical/surgical assistant	Counsellor	Clinic/community-based educator	Manager
General family planning					
Rationale for family planning, including female sterilization: health benefits; individual rights to determine family size; social, economic, and demographic concerns	XX	XX	XX	XX	XX
Status of family planning, including female sterilization: law and policies; cultural and religious factors; knowledge, attitudes and practices of family planning; availability of services; service goals and objectives	X	X	XX	XX	XX
Currently available temporary and permanent methods of family planning: how they work; effectiveness; advantages and disadvantages; risks and benefits	XX	XX	XX	XX	XX
Reproductive anatomy and physiology: applied anatomy and physiology of female and male reproductive systems; conception and pregnancy; general principles and effects of sterilization	XX	XX	XX	X	X
Free and informed choice					
General principles: client's right to choose any method or none; absence of coercion, inducements, pressure or					

misinformation; knowledge of characteristics, risks, and benefits of all methods; right to change mind at any time	XX	XX	XX	XX	XX
Counselling: client eligibility criteria; assessing the client's knowledge, decision-making, and preparedness for ending fertility; interactive and communicating skills; indicators of potential regret	XX	X	XX	X	X
Informed consent: meaning of informed consent; informed-consent form; process for obtaining informed consent; literate versus illiterate clients	X	X	XX	X	X
Community information and outreach					
Community and client information: techniques for providing general information to the community about sterilization and the location of services; interpersonal communication about sterilization in the community, hospitals, and service sites; client referral procedures				XX	X
Clinical support					
Clinic management: client registration; record-keeping; organization of clinic facilities and services; client flow	X	XX			X
Client instructions: preoperative and postoperative instructions to clients	XX	XX	XX	XX	X

Table 21. (cont.)

Knowledge, skills, and specific topics	Surgeon	Clinical/surgical assistant	Counsellor	Clinic/community-based educator	Manager
Asepsis, prevention of infection, and maintenance of equipment: basic hygiene; cleaning the facility; aseptic procedure; disinfection or sterilization of instruments and equipment; isolation of treatment and surgical areas	XX	XX			X
Medical and surgical procedures					
Preoperative patient evaluation: medical history; basic physical examination; pelvic examination; laboratory tests; contraindications	XX	XX	X		X
Preparing for surgery: preparing the operating theatre, equipment, and instruments; personnel requirements; preparing the client	XX	XX			X
Anaesthesia and client monitoring: types of anaesthesia; risks and benefits; indications and contraindications; monitoring and recording of vital signs; management of complications of anaesthesia	XX	XX	X		X
Surgical procedure: surgical approaches; techniques of tubal occlusion in relation to the timing of the procedure; surgical technique; complications and their management; assisting the surgeon; importance of teamwork	XX	XX	X		X

Emergency preparedness: emergency equipment (including manual resuscitator) and drugs; management of life-threatening complications; back-up systems	XX	XX			X
Postoperative care and follow-up examination: postoperative monitoring; postoperative instructions; basic follow-up examination, including removal of sutures; management of complications; assessment of client satisfaction	XX	XX	X		X
Management					
Planning: planning techniques; budgeting; staffing; community liaison					XX
Administration: clinic management; equipment and supply logistics; financial management; problem-solving		X			XX
Supervision: monitoring and supervision of service sites; recruitment, supervision, and assessment of personnel	X	X			XX
Evaluation: basic evaluation principles; record-keeping and reporting; service statistics and management information systems; assessment of performance, impact, and quality of services					XX

[a] The symbols "X" and "XX" are used to indicate which personnel require basic training, and which require advanced training in each specific topic.

to be trained. The specific criteria may also be influenced by local circumstances. Issues to be addressed in developing trainee selection criteria include minimum educational and professional qualifications, personal commitment, aptitude, and attitude. Also important is a commitment from the trainee's employing agency to allow the trainee to use his or her new skills, and to assign the trainee where those skills will be needed and can be used.

Evaluation and certification of trainees

Trainers must assess trainees continuously during training and must certify whether they have mastered the knowledge and skills required in order to work without direct supervision. Standard evaluation criteria for certification should be established for each category of personnel. In this regard, the World Federation of Health Agencies for the Advancement of Voluntary Surgical Contraception recommends that surgical trainees should perform a minimum of 10 solo minilaparotomies, 15 solo closed laparoscopies, or 10 solo open laparoscopies under direct supervision (WFHAAVSC, 1986 and 1988). Training may need to be extended for those trainees who, in the trainer's judgement, have not mastered the necessary knowledge and skills. A certificate of competence should be given only to those trainees who complete the programme requirements and whom the trainer assesses as competent to use their new skills without direct supervision.

Follow-up of trainees

Every training programme should also incorporate a system for routine follow-up of trainees. If possible, the trainers should conduct follow-up procedures in person at the home institutions of the trainees. Follow-up of trainees serves a number of important functions: it allows the trainee's performance to be evaluated; it offers an opportunity to correct deficiencies in knowledge and skills, as well as to provide encouragement and support; it assists in monitoring adherence to service standards and helps to identify areas where standards need to be changed; and it gives trainers an opportunity to identify weaknesses in the training curriculum. While personal, on-site follow-up of trainees is preferred, under some circumstances follow-up can be done through the use of questionnaires and workshops.

Resources for training programmes

The Association for Voluntary Surgical Contraception provides technical assistance and grants to assist institutions in establishing training programmes for personnel involved with female sterilization services. In addition, a number of other international family planning organizations specialize in training. Furthermore, many countries have developed high-quality training programmes for providers of female sterilization services that can serve as models and training sites. The addresses of some of these agencies are listed in Annex 1.

18. Monitoring and evaluation[1]

Monitoring and evaluation are often treated as separate aspects of management. However, they are closely related activities that help the service manager to determine whether guidelines and policies are being followed, whether objectives are being met, and whether problems are being recognized and addressed. Monitoring is the term used for the continuous follow-up of activities to ensure that they are proceeding according to plan. For example, it keeps track of the number of procedures performed, staff activities and performance, training, supplies and equipment, and the money spent in relation to the resources available, so that if anything goes wrong immediate corrective measures can be taken. Information gained from monitoring is used for evaluation. Evaluation is the systematic assessment of the relevance, adequacy, progress, effectiveness, and impact of a particular course of action. Effective systems for monitoring and evaluation are essential to ensure that services are proceeding as planned.

Setting relevant goals and objectives

Monitoring and evaluation can only be carried out in relation to specific goals and objectives. For female sterilization services, these goals and objectives fall into three general categories: medical safety and effectiveness, free and informed choice, and availability and accessibility of services.

Medical safety and effectiveness

All sterilization services should be safe and effective: efforts are needed to ensure that rates of complications, postoperative pain,

[1] For a general introduction to the theory and practice of monitoring and evaluation, see Korten & Korten, 1977; McMahon et al., 1980; Reynolds et al., 1978; and WHO, 1981.

and sterilization failures resulting in pregnancies are kept to a minimum. Every sterilization service should establish standards relating to medical safety; these should be followed by all service providers, and included in training. Experience in other countries can assist services in establishing standards for monitoring and evaluating medical safety and effectiveness. For example, experience in a number of countries suggests that about 0.5–1.0% of sterilizations fail, and that fewer than 10 deaths per 100 000 procedures are directly attributable to female sterilization. Therefore, if local rates are higher than these, service managers should take immediate corrective measures. In any case, every death associated with sterilization must be thoroughly investigated.

Free and informed choice

All clients must be given accurate information about female sterilization and understand the essential nature and effects of the procedure before making a decision. This decision should be made voluntarily, as discussed in Chapter 7. Furthermore, every client must have knowledge of and be able to obtain alternative, temporary methods of contraception.

Just as they establish standards for medical safety, all service and training programmes should develop guidelines and standard procedures to ensure that the client's choice is free and informed, and they should ensure that all personnel involved in planning and providing services are aware of the existence of these standards. Some indicators that can be monitored to determine whether the client's choice is being compromised are: complaints by clients that they were misinformed or coerced; the number of requests for reversal; the availability and clients' knowledge of temporary methods of family planning; the adequacy of client counselling; and the accuracy of reports about female sterilization in the mass media and among service providers.

Availability and accessibility

Ensuring that voluntary sterilization and other contraceptive methods are available and easily accessible to all potential clients should be a long-term goal of family planning services. Evidence of progress towards this goal would be an increase in prevalence of contraceptive practice, including reliance on sterilization; reductions in maternal morbidity and mortality as more women choose sterilization; and a reduction in the number of births to high-parity, older women and others at high risk. Over the shorter term, managers need to have a clear, quantified plan of action relating to the number of personnel to be trained, service sites to be established, and the expected case-load. Indicators for assessing the availability and accessibility of family planning services include: the number and location of service sites; the availability of adequate supplies and equipment; the number and characteristics of clients undergoing sterilization; the number, type, and distribution of trained service personnel; and the costs of services.

Making appropriate and timely observations

Once the goals and objectives are clearly defined, managers need to develop schemes for monitoring and evaluation of services. The service manager, or director of services, should ensure that adequate time, attention, and resources are apportioned to these activities. Different types of activity are required according to the nature and urgency of the monitoring and evaluation needed. Services should have the capacity to address three situations:

- Special *urgent investigations* to deal with serious events or problems of compelling importance.
- *Routine monitoring* to collect basic management information about performance.
- *Special research and studies* occasionally undertaken to investigate or assess particular issues, problems, or questions.

The application of these different types of activity to sterilization services is outlined in Table 22 and is discussed in further detail below.

Urgent investigations

Service directors (i.e., senior managers) must be aware of and respond promptly to any serious problems associated with medical care or free and informed choice. Examples of serious medical safety problems are deaths attributable to sterilization, life-threatening complications of surgery, and high rates of complications or sterilization failures. Possibly serious problems related to free and informed choice include reports of involuntary or coerced sterilization, the provision of misleading information about sterilization at a service site or in the mass media, reported high rates of regret or requests for reversal, and sudden, sharp increases in the number of sterilizations, which might be a response to coercive or misleading practices. While such problems may be relatively rare events, they must be investigated urgently

Table 22. Monitoring and evaluating voluntary sterilization services

	Major concerns		
Type of activity	Medical safety and effectiveness	Free and informed choice	Availability and accessibility
Urgent investigations	Fatalities Serious complications High rates of complications and failures	Involuntary sterilization A sudden, sharp rise in the number of clients High rates of regret and requests for reversal Misleading information activities	A sudden, unexplained fall in the number of clients
Routine monitoring (via direct observation or data collection and reporting systems)	Clinical services management Surgical skills and medical practices Number and types of complications and failures	Counselling practices and skills Informed-consent procedures Number of and reasons for requests for reversal Number of and reasons for client rejection Availability of alternative temporary methods of contraception	Number and types of procedures Characteristics of clients (e.g., age, parity) Number and location of service sites and trained personnel Logistics and cash flow

Table 22. (cont.)

Type of activity	Major concerns: Medical safety and effectiveness	Major concerns: Free and informed choice	Major concerns: Availability and accessibility
Special research and studies	Clinical studies or trials of technological innovations and surgical techniques Surveys of clinical or surgical practices	Surveys and studies of satisfaction among clients Knowledge, attitudes and practices of clients Client decision-making studies Incentives and disincentives	Prevalence surveys Cost studies Information programmes Attitudes of personnel Operations research aimed at improving services

because their occurrence may indicate serious lapses in adherence to service standards. If left unattended, these problems are likely to recur, the health and rights of clients may be further abused and the reputation of the female sterilization service is likely to be severely, perhaps irreparably, damaged.

Procedures for investigating every death related to sterilization should be established for every service-delivery site (WFHAAVSC, 1988). Deaths may be detected through established reporting systems or via sources other than the service provider, such as family members, clinic staff, other health providers, or the media. Service managers should give such reports prompt attention to assess whether the death resulted from the procedure, to identify all of the possible contributing factors, and to take effective action. Senior doctors who are familiar with major medical complications associated with sterilization should also be available to review carefully all the details surrounding the case. Usually recommendations are then made for practices to be changed at the clinic involved or at all service sites in order to reduce the chances of further deaths. The service director should be aware that some deaths are likely to occur.

The service director, usually in conjunction with the senior medical staff, must be prepared to review the findings of any investigation into a death and take corrective action to reduce the chances of a recurrence. Each death is a highly sensitive issue for the family, the medical staff directly involved, and the community. In acquiring the necessary information and implementing any recommendations, great care must be taken to respect confidentiality, to avoid creating any additional problems for the family, and to maintain the credibility of the service.

Reports of high numbers of complications or failures should also be assessed by medical supervisory staff through an on-site review to confirm that a problem exists and to identify the potential causes. The urgency of this investigation will depend on the severity and frequency of the complications and the number of failures reported. Sometimes these problems are restricted to one particular practitioner or clinic. Occasionally they may indicate a more extensive problem that needs wider attention and corrective action, such as a change in guidelines or training practices.

As with any serious medical problem, reports of involuntary sterilization or other breaches of free and informed choice require direct investigation by the manager or by other qualified, senior personnel. The service manager should determine whether the lapse was an isolated occurrence that might necessitate special technical assistance or retraining of local service personnel, or whether it indicates more extensive underlying problems that might require changes in policies, service standards, or routine practices. Corrective action should be taken at the local site in collaboration with local personnel, and the service manager should ensure that any recommendations are implemented.

Routine monitoring

All health and family planning services should have routine systems for the regular monitoring of services. These generally involve two complementary methods of observation: collecting and analysing service statistics and other data through management information systems; and making direct observations, usually through scheduled and unscheduled visits to local service sites by supervisors. Some of the concerns of routine monitoring are listed in Table 22.

Ideally, routine monitoring of voluntary sterilization services should be integrated with the monitoring of other health and family planning services. For example, data relating to the number and type of sterilization procedures performed can be included in the monthly reports of family planning services. If female sterilization services are monitored independently, this may be more expensive, more demanding of local staff, and more difficult to sustain in the long term. Nevertheless, given the special character of sterilization services, some additional routine monitoring activities may be required, especially when services are being introduced and greater attention is required.

Routine monitoring may involve a separate system in which the doctor is responsible for recording and reporting any complications to a central facility. Such formal surveillance systems are useful for establishing definitions and criteria for complications. They can indicate which are the most common types of complications, but they may be limited in their ability to identify specific clinics or practices associated with a higher risk of complications or failures. This is partly because complications are generally underreported. It is also difficult to maintain an effective independent reporting system in the long term without involving considerable expense and effort.

Much of the information that is required for routine monitoring of services can be derived from the medical record forms of sterilization clients. Services sometimes develop a standard medical record form for sterilization procedures to ensure that all the necessary clinical and surgical details are available for each client. This form also serves as a reminder to staff to perform certain duties. It also provides the basis for investigating any complications or deaths. Guidelines for developing a medical record form designed for female sterilization services are given in Annex 5, together with an example of a typical form.

Some services find it useful to compile summary reports of certain details taken from the medical record forms of all clients who were served during a particular period. This is sometimes done monthly (see Annex 5). This report allows service managers, at local and central levels, to review quickly all the procedures performed during a given period, in order to identify unusual occurrences or trends in services that require further investigation. Information from this report can also help to identify weaknesses in medical care, personnel, or skills that can be addressed by additional training. However, since this type of report involves extra time and effort, it should be required only if service managers are trained in how to interpret and use it.

Additional qualitative assessments of local services involving direct observation are required to supplement statistical reporting systems. These often involve scheduled (and sometimes unscheduled) visits to local service sites by doctors, nurses, or other supervisory or technical personnel. These visits may be used to observe practices and assess adherence to established guidelines on medical safety, counselling, and other aspects of service delivery. For example, they may include observation and discussion of medical practices, surgical technique, clinic cleanliness and asepsis, record-keeping, counselling and informed consent, and treatment of clients. Visiting supervisors should talk to both clinic staff and clients. In addition, they should encourage all staff involved in providing services to assess their own work continually.

Special research and studies

In addition to the routine and continuous monitoring of basic service statistics, special research and studies are sometimes required to investigate particular issues, problems, or questions to make more refined analyses of trends detected during routine data collection or to modify service design for better results. In general, however, only a limited number of such studies should be conducted, since they can be more expensive and take up more time than routine activities, and may involve skills that are not available locally, thus requiring outside technical advisors.

On the other hand, local service managers are usually able to conduct (or can arrange for others to conduct) non-routine studies or investigations that are relatively simple, quick to perform, and inexpensive. For example, they might occasionally interview a small sample of clients after surgery to learn how clients perceive the services and to identify problems in their treatment by staff. Alternatively, they might contact a sample of clients who fail to show up for their appointments, to learn the reasons. These investigations can provide local managers with considerable insights.

Some examples of these studies are briefly discussed below and in Table 22.

Client satisfaction. A major area of concern for all sterilization services is the degree to which clients are satisfied with the service and the sterilization procedure. Dissatisfaction among clients may be related to factors that can be controlled by reviewing and redesigning services. Methods that may be used to assess client satisfaction include surveys, focus groups, in-depth interviews, and informal, ad hoc investigations by local service managers.

Availability and accessibility of services. Limited availability and accessibility of services can be a major obstacle to clients. Several factors may be involved: policies and regulations about age, parity, and spousal consent; attitudes of service-delivery personnel; the number, location, staffing, and timing of services; the type of service-delivery channels, institutions, and sectors involved; and the procedures clients must follow to obtain a sterilization. Studies of these factors can provide important information for planning or modifying services.

Knowledge and attitudes of clients, providers, and the community. Assessing client knowledge and attitudes about sterilization can be important in identifying fears, misinformation, rumours, and other negative influences on acceptance of sterilization. After identifying such factors, service managers can design information strategies to correct false impressions and negative attitudes (see Chapter 6). Because health providers sometimes oppose or resist sterilization services, it is important to assess their knowledge and attitudes as well as those of potential clients. This information can be obtained through surveys, focus group discussions, and interviews. Questions can also be included in surveys of fertility or contraceptive prevalence. In addition, local service managers may occasionally conduct informal ad hoc interviews with clients and community leaders to assess the knowledge and attitudes of the community.

Cost. Insufficient information is available about the total costs of delivering sterilization services or about the cost-effectiveness of alternative delivery systems. Cost studies can be difficult and expensive, but they are essential to determine the most efficient service designs, especially if funding is limited and services are unable to recover costs directly from clients or through other means.

Incentives and disincentives. Another important study area is the use of payments to clients or providers and other incentives and disincentives (see pages 75–76). If payments or benefits are given, their influence on the client's request for sterilization and on the provider should be examined. The cost-effectiveness and social effects of providing incentives and disincentives should also be explored.

Improving the effectiveness of monitoring and evaluation

It is generally agreed that systems for routine monitoring of female sterilization services should be kept as simple as possible, since this will increase the likelihood of such systems being sustained over the long term. If service-delivery systems involve excessive data collection and reporting, or numerous visits by supervisors, they may not function effectively (WHO, 1989a).

Systems for monitoring and evaluation of sterilization services should be integrated, as far as is practicable, with existing monitoring and evaluation systems for other family planning and health services. This reduces costs by making use of available staff and resources, and increases the likelihood of the systems being sustained. It also reduces intrusion on client and staff time. However, specific systems may need to be established when services are being introduced or when particular aspects or problems associated with sterilization services are being examined.

Furthermore, training activities should be closely linked with monitoring and evaluation. Any problems or deviations from standard practices detected through monitoring and evaluation can often be addressed through initial, refresher, and in-service training.

In addition, monitoring and evaluation activities should be executed in a timely manner to ensure that services proceed as planned, to maintain the quality of services, to reduce the likelihood of any problems occurring, and to minimize any problems that do occur.

Furthermore, service managers should not rely solely on these formal systems and procedures to collect information and make observations. Other sources such as their personal intuition, chance observations, and independent (non-service) sources may provide important information that would not be obtained by the formal systems, and they may offer a different perspective on services.

Service managers should recognize that systems for monitoring and evaluation of services will need to be developed and modified concurrently with the services themselves. The extent and complexity of such systems will vary between countries, depending on local conditions, as well as at different times within a given service. For example, the service manager may need to adopt an extensive, active, and formal monitoring system when services are being introduced or expanded to new localities, when a new surgical technique or service management procedure is widely introduced, or when major staff changes occur. The system can then be modified once the manager is satisfied that the innovations or changes are functioning well.

Monitoring and evaluation should also support and benefit local personnel. If local personnel are required to participate in the systems—for example, by being observed by supervisors, or collecting data and submitting routine reports—they should receive feedback on the findings from managers and supervisors. The systems should not impose unreasonable burdens on local service personnel and should respect their limited time and busy schedules. The trust and cooperation of local staff are essential. If staff fear the results of monitoring and evaluation, they may not cooperate. Therefore, systems should always be designed and used in ways that are non-threatening and non-punitive.

References

ALTOBELLI, L. C. ET AL. (1980a) *Advanced laparoscopic systems: preventive care and maintenance*. Baltimore, Johns Hopkins Program for International Education in Gynecology and Obstetrics.

ALTOBELLI, L. C. ET AL. (1980b) *Laprocator: preventive care and maintenance*. Baltimore, Johns Hopkins Program for International Education in Gynecology and Obstetrics.

ANGLE, M. ET AL. (1989) *Sterilization, disinfection, decontamination, and cleaning of FP/MCH clinic equipment*. Chapel Hill, NC, Program for International Training in Health.

ASSOCIATION FOR VOLUNTARY SURGICAL CONTRACEPTION (forthcoming) *Sterilization reversal: issues and implications for voluntary surgical contraception*. New York.

BHIWANDIWALA, P. P. ET AL. (1982) A comparison of different laparoscopic sterilization occlusion techniques in 24,439 procedures. *American journal of obstetrics and gynecology*, **144**(3): 319–331.

BORING, C. C. ET AL. (1988) Sterilization regret among Puerto Rican women. *Fertility and sterility*, **49** (6): 973–981.

BUTTA, P. (1988) *Informed consent and voluntary surgical contraception*. New York, Association for Voluntary Surgical Contraception.

CALLAGHAN, P. (1986) Hands off the peritoneum. *Lancet*, **1** (8485): 849–850.

CHATURACHINDA, K. (1976) Minilaparotomy and laparoscopy. In: Schima, M. E. & Lubell, I., eds. *New advances in sterilization*. New York, Association for Voluntary Sterilization.

CHENG, M. C. E. ET AL. (1977) Sterilization failures in Singapore: an examination of ligation techniques and failure rates. *Studies in family planning*, **8** (4): 109–115.

CHI, I.-C. ET AL. (1980) An epidemiologic study of risk factors associated with pregnancy following female sterilization. *American journal of obstetrics and gynecology*, **136** (6): 768–773.

CHI, I.-C. ET AL. (1981) Pregnancy risk following laparoscopic sterilization in nongravid and gravid women. *Journal of reproductive medicine*, **26** (6): 289–294.

CHOWDHURY, S. & CHOWDHURY, Z. (1975) Tubectomy by paraprofessional surgeons in rural Bangladesh. *Lancet*, **2** (7935): 567–569.

COOK, J. ET AL., ed. (1991) *Surgery at the district hospital: obstetrics, gynaecology, orthopaedics, and traumatology*. Geneva, World Health Organization.

CUMMINS, G. T. M. (1976) An overview of female sterilization. In: Schima, M. E. & Lubell, I., eds. *New advances in sterilization*. New York, Association for Voluntary Sterilization.

DARNEY, P. D., ed. (1987) *Handbook of office and ambulatory gynecologic surgery*. Oradell, NJ, Medical Economics.

DESTEFANO, F. ET AL. (1982) Risk of ectopic pregnancy following tubal sterilization. *Obstetrics and gynecology*, **60** (3): 326–330.

DESTEFANO, F. ET AL. (1983) Complications of interval laparoscopic tubal sterilization. *Obstetrics and gynecology*, **61** (2): 153–158.

DOBSON, M. B. (1988) *Anaesthesia at the district hospital*. Geneva, World Health Organization.

EDMUNDS, M. ET AL. (1987) *Client-responsive family planning: a handbook for providers*. Watertown, MA, Pathfinder Fund.

FISHBURNE, J. I. (1981) *A report on a consultation to the Bangladesh Association for Voluntary Sterilization*. Washington, DC, United States Agency for International Development.

FISHBURNE, J. I. (1983) Anesthesia for outpatient female sterilization. *Biomedical bulletin*, **4** (1): 1–6.

FISHBURNE, J. I. & KEITH, L. (1977) Anesthesia. In: Phillips, J. M., ed. *Laparoscopy*. Baltimore, Williams and Wilkins.

GILLESPIE, D. G. ET AL. (1988) *Financing the delivery of contraceptives: the challenge of the next twenty years*. Washington, DC, United States Agency for International Development.

GRIMES, D. A. ET AL. (1982) Sterilization-attributable deaths in Bangladesh. *International journal of obstetrics and gynaecology*, **20**: 149–154.

HASSON, H. M. (1982) Open laparoscopy. In: Sciarra, J. J., ed. *Gynecology and obstetrics*. Philadelphia, Harper & Row.

HASSON, H. M. (1984) Open laparoscopy. *Biomedical bulletin*, **5** (1): 1–6.

HATCHER, R. A. ET AL. (1988) *Contraceptive technology 1988–1989*. Atlanta, Printed Matter.

HATCHER, R. A. ET AL. (1989) *Contraceptive technology: international edition*. Atlanta, Printed Matter.

HENRY, A. ET AL. (1980) Reversing female sterilization. *Population reports*, Series C, No. 8.

HUBER, D. H. (1989) Voluntary surgical contraception (sterilization). In: Hatcher, R. A. et al. *Contraceptive technology: international edition*. Atlanta, Printed Matter.

HUBER, D. H. ET AL. (1989) *Characteristics of clips for female sterilization*. Paper presented at Second World Congress of Endoscopic Female Sterilization, Williamsburg, Virginia, United States, 9–12 July 1987.[1]

---

[1] Unpublished document; available on request from the Association for Voluntary Surgical Contraception, 79 Madison Avenue, New York, NY 10016, USA.

HUBER, S. C. & HARVEY, P. D. (1989) Family planning programmes in the developing countries. *Journal of biosocial science*, **21** (3): 267–277.

HULKA, J. F. & HALME, J. (1988) Sterilization reversal: results of 101 attempts. *American journal of obstetrics and gynecology*, **159** (3): 767–774.

HUNT, R. B. (1986) *Atlas of female infertility survey*. Chicago, Year Book Medical Publishers.

INDIAN COUNCIL OF MEDICAL RESEARCH (1982) *Collaborative study on sequelae of tubal sterilization*. New Delhi.

ISAACS, S. L. & COOK, R. J. (1984) Laws and policies affecting fertility: a decade of change. *Population reports*, Series E, No. 7.

JEZOWSKI, T. W. & ELLIS, A. (1987) *Assessment of the institutionalization of family planning and voluntary surgical contraception services in Nepal: report submitted to His Majesty's government of Nepal and the U.S. Agency for International Development*. New York, Association for Voluntary Surgical Contraception.

JONES, E. F. & FORREST, J. D. (1989) Contraceptive failure in the United States: revised estimates from the 1982 National Survey of Family Growth. *Family planning perspectives*, **21** (3): 103–109.

KING, M., ed. (1986) *Primary anaesthesia*. Oxford, Oxford University Press.

KORTEN, F. F. & KORTEN, D. C. (1977) *Casebook for family planning management: motivating effective clinic performance*. Chestnut Hill, MA, Pathfinder Fund.

KWAK, H. M. (1987) Laparoscopic sterilizations: Korean experience, particularly ectopic pregnancy subsequent to female sterilizations. In: *Proceedings of the Pre-Congress Seminar of the XIth AOFOG Congress, Bangkok, Thailand, December 1–4, 1987*. Asia and Oceania Federation of Obstetrics and Gynecology.

LISKIN, L. ET AL. (1985) Minilaparotomy and laparoscopy: safe, effective, and widely used. *Population reports*, Series C, No. 9.

MAINE, D. (1981) *Family planning: its impact on the health of women and children*. New York, Center for Population and Family Health, Columbia University.

MARCIL-GRATTON, N. (1988) Sterilization regret among women in metropolitan Montreal. *Family planning perspectives*, **20** (5): 222–227.

MAULDIN, W. P. & SEGAL, S. J. (1988) Prevalence of contraceptive use: trends and issues. *Studies in family planning*, **19** (6): 335–353.

MCBRIDE, M. ET AL. (1987) Cost-effectiveness of the APROFAM program for voluntary surgical contraception in Guatemala. *Evaluation review*, **11** (3): 300–326.

MCCANN, M. F. (1978) Laparoscopy versus minilaparotomy. In: Sciarra, J. J. et al., eds. *Risks, benefits, and controversies in fertility control*. Hagerstown, MD, Harper & Row.

MCFADDEN, P. M. & PEACOCK, E. E., JR. (1983) Preperitoneal abdominal wound repair: incidence of dehiscence. *American journal of surgery*, **145**: 213–214.

McMahon, R. et al. (1992) *On being in charge: a guide to management in primary health care*, 2nd ed. Geneva, World Health Organization.

Moss, W. M. & Association for Voluntary Surgical Contraception (1988) *Contraceptive sterilization.* Amityville, NY, Essential Medical Information Systems.

Mumford, S. D. & Bhiwandiwala, P. P. (1981) Tubal ring sterilization: experience with 10,086 cases. *Obstetrics and gynecology*, **57** (2): 150–157.

Mumford, S. D. et al. (1980) Laparoscopic and minilaparotomy female sterilization compared in 15,167 cases. *Lancet*, **2** (8203): 1066–1070.

Neamatalla, G. S. & Harper, P. B. (1990) *Family planning counseling and voluntary sterilization: a guide for managers.* New York, Association for Voluntary Surgical Contraception.

Penfield, A. J. (1980) *Female sterilization by minilaparotomy or open laparoscopy.* Baltimore, Urban & Schwarzenberg.

Peterson, H. B. et al. (1983) Deaths attributable to tubal sterilization in the United States, 1977 to 1981. *American journal of obstetrics and gynecology*, **146** (2): 131–136.

Philliber, S. G. & Philliber, W. W. (1985) Social and psychological perspectives on voluntary sterilization: a review. *Studies in family planning*, **16** (1): 1–29.

Phillips, J. M. (1981) *Microsurgery in gynecology II.* Downey, CA, American Association of Gynecologic Laparoscopists.

Population Communication Services & Population Information Program (date not known) *Basic processes and principles for population/family planning communication.* Baltimore, Johns Hopkins University.

Porter, C. W., jr. (1987) Prevention of infection in voluntary surgical contraception. *Biomedical bulletin*, **6** (1): 1–7.

Pritchard, J. A. et al. (1985) *Williams obstetrics*, 17th ed. Norwalk, CT, Appleton-Century-Crofts.

Program for Appropriate Technology in Health (1988) *Overview of the materials development process.* Washington, DC.

Puffer, R. R. & Serrano, C. V. (1975) *Birthweight, maternal age, and birth order: three important determinants of infant mortality.* Washington, DC, Pan American Health Organization (Scientific Publication No. 294).

Reynolds, J. et al. (1978) *Evaluation handbook for family planning programmes.* Rockville, MD, United States Department of Health, Education, and Welfare.

Rock, J. A. et al. (1982) Tubal anastomosis following unipolar cautery. *Fertility and sterility*, **37** (5): 613–618.

Rogers, E. M. (1973) *Communication strategies for family planning.* New York, Free Press.

Ross, J. A. et al. (1985) *Voluntary sterilization: an international fact book.* New York, Association for Voluntary Sterilization.

Ross, J. A. et al. (1988) *Family planning and child survival: 100 developing countries.* New York, Center for Population and Family Health, Columbia University.

Ross, J. A. et al. (1989) *Management strategies for family planning programs.* New York, Center for Population and Family Health, Columbia University.

Satyapan, S. et al. (1983) Postpartum tubal ligation by nurse-midwives in Thailand: a field trial. *Studies in family planning,* **14**(4): 115–118.

Sciarra, J. J. et al. (1978) *Reversal of sterilization.* Hagerstown, MD, Harper & Row.

Spivak, M. M. et al. (1986) Microsurgical reversal of sterilization: a six-year study. *American journal of obstetrics and gynecology,* **154**(2): 355–361.

Starrs, A. (1987) *Preventing the tragedy of maternal deaths: a report on the International Safe Motherhood Conference.* Washington, DC, World Bank.

Stewart, F. et al. (1987) *Understanding your body.* Toronto, Bantam.

Tietjen, L. G. & McIntosh, N. (1989) Infection control in family planning facilities. *Outlook,* **7**(2): 2–8.

Trussell, J. & Kost, K. (1987) Contraceptive failure in the United States: a critical review of the literature. *Studies in family planning,* **18**(5): 237–283.

United Nations Fund for Population Activities (1985) *UNFPA assistance and population data* (wall chart). New York.

Vessey, M. et al. (1983) Tubal sterilization: findings in a large prospective study. *British journal of obstetrics and gynaecology,* **90**(3): 203–209.

WFHAAVSC (1983) *Standard terms for voluntary surgical contraception.* New York, World Federation of Health Agencies for the Advancement of Voluntary Surgical Contraception.

WFHAAVSC (1984) *Safety of voluntary surgical contraception.* New York, World Federation of Health Agencies for the Advancement of Voluntary Surgical Contraception.

WFHAAVSC (1986) *Training guidelines for voluntary surgical contraception.* New York, World Federation of Health Agencies for the Advancement of Voluntary Surgical Contraception.

WFHAAVSC (1987) *Voluntary choice and surgical contraception.* New York, World Federation of Health Agencies for the Advancement of Voluntary Surgical Contraception.

WFHAAVSC (1988) *Safe and voluntary surgical contraception.* New York, World Federation of Health Agencies for the Advancement of Voluntary Surgical Contraception.

Wheeless, C. R. & Katayama, K. P. (1985) Laparoscopy and tubal sterilization. In: Mattingly, R. F. & Thompson, J. D., eds. *Te Linde's operative gynecology.* Philadelphia, Lippincott.

WHO (1981) *Health programme evaluation: guiding principles for its application in the managerial process for national health development.* Geneva, World Health Organization.

WHO (1989a) Experts call for medical monitoring and supervision of sterilization services. *Progress*, No. 10: 4.

WHO (1989b) *Guidelines on sterilization and disinfection methods effective against human immunodeficiency virus (HIV)*, 2nd ed. Geneva, World Health Organization (WHO AIDS Series 2).

WHO (1989) *WHO model prescribing information: drugs used in anaesthesia.* Geneva, World Health Organization.

WHO Task Force on Female Sterilization (1982a) Mini-incision for postpartum sterilization of women: a multicentered, multinational prospective study. *Contraception*, **26** (5): 495–503.

WHO Task Force on Female Sterilization (1982b) Minilaparotomy or laparoscopy for sterilization: a multicenter, multinational randomized study. *American journal of obstetrics and gynecology*, **143** (6): 645–652.

WHO Task Force on Female Sterilization (1982c) Randomized comparative study of culdoscopy and minilaparotomy for surgical contraception in women. *Contraception*, **26** (6): 587–593.

Whong, Y. W. (1987) *Ectopic pregnancy subsequent to female sterilization.* Seoul, Korean Association for Voluntary Sterilization.

Wimberley, E. T. & Abplanalp, J. M. (1983) Poststerilization regret among women: methodological considerations for the next decade. *Biomedical bulletin*, **4** (2): 1–6 .

Zatuchni, G. I. et al. (1983) *Female transcervical sterilization.* Philadelphia, Harper & Row.

Zimmerman, M. L. & Perkin, G. W. (1982) *Print materials for nonreaders: experiences in family planning and health.* Seattle, Program for the Introduction and Adaptation of Contraceptive Technology (PIACT Paper No. 8).

Additional sources of information

AMERICAN COLLEGE OF OBSTETRICIANS AND GYNECOLOGISTS (1988) Sterilization. *ACOG Technical Bulletin*, No. 113.

ASSOCIATION FOR VOLUNTARY SURGICAL CONTRACEPTION (1987) *Report on voluntarism workshop*. New York.

BUTTA, P. ET AL. (1987) Protecting voluntary, informed choice. *AVSC news*, **25**(4): 4, 6.

DUSITSIN, N. & SATAYAPAN, S. (1984) Sterilization of women by nurse-midwives in Thailand. *World health forum*, **5**(3): 259–262.

FADEN, R. R. ET AL. (1986) *A history of informed consent*. New York, Oxford University Press.

FAMILY PLANNING ASSOCIATION OF KENYA & ASSOCIATION FOR VOLUNTARY SURGICAL CONTRACEPTION (1989) *Counselling: helping people make family planning choices* (film/video). Nairobi and New York.

FAMILY PLANNING ASSOCIATION OF KENYA & ASSOCIATION FOR VOLUNTARY SURGICAL CONTRACEPTION (1989) *Minilaparotomy for voluntary surgical contraception* (film/video). Nairobi and New York.

FRITZ, L. (1992) *Equipment for VSC programs: a manual for AVSC staff*. New York, Association for Voluntary Surgical Contraception.

GALLEN, M. ET AL. (1987) Counseling makes a difference. *Population reports*, Series J, No. 35.

HAALAND, A. (1984) *Pretesting communication materials*. Rangoon, United Nations Children's Fund.

HOLTROP, H. R. & WAIFE, R. S. (1978) *Minilaparotomy techniques*. Chestnut Hill, MA, Pathfinder Fund.

HUBER, D. H. *Medical and health aspects of voluntary surgical contraception*. Paper presented at Fifth International Conference on Voluntary Surgical Contraception, Santo Domingo, Dominican Republic, 5–8 December 1983.[1]

HUTCHINGS, J. & SAUNDERS, L. (1985) *Assessing the characteristics and cost-effectiveness of contraceptive methods*. Seattle, Program for the Introduction and Adaptation of Contraceptive Technology (PIACT Paper No. 10).

[1] Unpublished document; available on request from the Association for Voluntary Surgical Contraception, 79 Madison Avenue, New York, NY 10016, USA.

ISAACS, S. L. *Informed consent for family planning: an analysis of the legal and ethical issues.* Paper presented at meeting of the American Public Health Association, Dallas, Texas, USA, 13–17 November 1983.[1]

JAIN, A. K. (1989) Fertility reduction and the quality of family planning services. *Studies in family planning*, **20** (1): 1–16.

JEZOWSKI, T. W. *The development of training capacity for the introduction of new contraceptive technology.* Paper presented at meeting of the American Public Health Association, Las Vegas, Nevada, USA, 29 September 1986.[1]

JEZOWSKI, T. W. *Quality assurance for voluntary sterilization.* Paper presented at Conference on Contraceptive Technology Update, Dhaka, Bangladesh, 2–3 November 1986.[1]

KLEINMAN, R. L., ed. (1982) *Female sterilization.* London, International Planned Parenthood Federation.

KLEINMAN, R. L., ed. (1988) *Family planning handbook for doctors.* London, International Planned Parenthood Federation.

KOETSAWANG, S. ET AL. (1981) Postpartum sterilization by operating-room nurses in Thailand. *International journal of gynaecology and obstetrics*, **19**: 201–204.

LANDRY, E. G. (1990) How and why women choose sterilization: results from six follow-up surveys. *Studies in family planning*, **21** (3): 143–151.

LAUFE, L. E. & MCCANN, M. F. (1978) Training: an integral adjunct to the introduction of newer methods of fertility regulation. *International journal of gynaecology and obstetrics*, **15**: 302–306.

LETTENMAIER, C. & GALLEN, M. E. (1987) Why counseling counts! *Population reports*, Series J, No. 36.

LISKIN, L. ET AL. (1983) Vasectomy: safe and simple. *Population reports*, Series D, No. 4.

PALMER, R. ET AL. (1987) *La stérilisation volontaire en France et dans le monde.* [*Voluntary sterilization in France and in the world.*] Paris, Masson.

PAN AMERICAN HEALTH ORGANIZATION (1984) *Guía para el diseño, utilización, y evaluación de materiales educativos de salud.* [*A guide for the design, use, and evaluation of health education material.*] Washington, DC.

PENFIELD, A. J. (1986) *Gynecologic surgery under local anesthesia.* Baltimore, Urban & Schwarzenberg.

PHILLIBER, S. G. (1988) *Contraception and informed choice in the United States.* Research Triangle Park, NC, Family Health International.

PHILLIPS, A. J. & D'ABLAING, G., III. (1986) Acute salpingitis subsequent to tubal ligation. *Obstetrics and gynecology*, **67** (3): 55S–58S.

PILE, J. M. (1988) *Background notes on sterilization reversal.* New York, World Federation of Health Agencies for the Advancement of Voluntary Surgical Contraception.

[1] Unpublished document; available on request from the Association for Voluntary Surgical Contraception, 79 Madison Avenue, New York, NY 10016, USA.

RAHMAN, A. & JEZOWSKI, T. J. (1983) Safer anesthesia practices introduced in VSC programs in Bangladesh. *Communiqué*, **4** (2): 6–7.

ROSENBERG, M. J. ET AL. (1982) Sterilization in Bangladesh: mortality, morbidity, and risk factors. *International journal of gynaecology and obstetrics*, **20**: 283–291.

RUBIN, G. L. ET AL. (1982) The mortality risk of voluntary surgical contraception. *Biomedical bulletin*, **3** (2): 1–5.

SATTERTHWAITE, A. P. (1981) *Study of sterilization-related deaths in Bangladesh from July 1, 1980 to April 15, 1989*. Dhaka, Institute of Population Research and Training, Government of Bangladesh.

TANG, G. W. K. & KWAN, M. (1988) Nonsurgical sterilization using phenol-mucilage: acceptability and efficacy. *Contraception*, **37** (6): 599–606.

UNITED STATES: DEPARTMENT OF HEALTH AND HUMAN SERVICES (1982) *Pretesting in health communications*. Bethesda, MD, Public Health Service, National Institutes of Health.

WFHAAVSC (1982) *Expansion of voluntary surgical contraception into rural, remote, and peripheral areas*. New York, World Federation of Health Agencies for the Advancement of Voluntary Surgical Contraception.

WFHAAVSC (1987) *Counseling and voluntary sterilization: a guide for family planning programs*. New York, World Federation of Health Agencies for the Advancement of Voluntary Surgical Contraception.

WHO (1988) *Technical and managerial guidelines for vasectomy services*. Geneva, World Health Organization.

ZIMMERMAN, M. L. (1982) Instructing through pictures. *Communiqué*, **3** (1): 3.

Annex 1. Sources of technical and funding assistance for female sterilization services

Agency	Principal type(s) of assistance
Association for Voluntary Surgical Contraception (AVSC) 79 Madison Avenue New York, NY 10016 USA	Grants and technical assistance for training, and provision of equipment and supplies to establish, expand, and improve voluntary sterilization services.
Centers for Disease Control (CDC) Division of Reproductive Health 1600 Clifton Road, N.W. Atlanta, GA 30333 USA	Technical assistance in management and evaluation of family planning programmes.
Family Health International (FHI) P.O. Box 13950 Research Triangle Park Branch Durham, NC 27709 USA	Support for clinical, epidemiological, and service-oriented research.
Family Planning Association of Kenya (FPAK) P.O. Box 30581, Harambee Plaza Haile Selassie Avenue Nairobi Kenya	Training in family planning counselling and in interval and postpartum female sterilization surgery using minilaparotomy.

Agency	Principal type(s) of assistance
International Planned Parenthood Federation (IPPF) Regent's College Inner Circle Regent's Park London NW1 4NS England	Grants, technical assistance, and equipment for service, training, and information programmes. Assistance is restricted primarily to IPPF affiliates.
The JHPIEGO Corporation (a Johns Hopkins Program for International Education in Reproductive Health) Brown's Wharf 1615 Thames Street Baltimore, MD 21231 USA	Specialized training for health professionals in medical and management skills for reproductive health care, including voluntary sterilization.
Maternidad Nuestra Señora de la Altagracia Calle Guarocuya No. 90 El Millon Santo Domingo Dominican Republic	Training in postpartum female sterilization surgery using minilaparotomy.
The Pathfinder Fund 9 Galen Street, Suite 217 Watertown, MA 02172 USA	Grants and equipment for service, training, and information programmes.
Population Communication Services (PCS) The Johns Hopkins University School of Hygiene and Public Health, Center for Communication Programs 527 St Paul Place Baltimore, MD 21202 USA	Grants and technical assistance for information programme development; mass media, print materials, and audiovisual materials.

Agency	Principal type(s) of assistance
The Population Council 1 Dag Hammarskjold Plaza New York, NY 10017 USA	Support for operations research and evaluation of services and training, and for contraceptive research.
The Program for Appropriate Technology in Health (PATH) 4 Nickerson Street Seattle, WA 98109 USA	Grants and technical assistance for development of information materials for family planning users and providers.
Program for International Training in Health (INTRAH) University of North Carolina 208 North Columbia Street Chapel Hill, NC 27514 USA	Grants, technical assistance, and equipment for training of family planning service providers.
The Philippines Association for Voluntary Surgical Contraception (PAVSC) 2nd Floor, IMCH Building 11 Banawe Street Quezon City, Manila Philippines	Training in counselling for family planning providers.
United Nations Population Fund (UNFPA) 220 East 42nd Street New York, NY 10017 USA	Support to government services, training programmes, and equipment procurement. In many countries, contact may be made directly through the UNFPA representative.

Agency	Principal type(s) of assistance
US Agency for International Development (USAID) Office of Population Science and Technology Bureau Washington, DC 20523 USA	Support to governments and cooperating agencies for family planning services, research, and provision of contraceptives. In many countries, contact may be made directly through the USAID Mission or American Embassy.
World Health Organization 20 Avenue Appia 1211 Geneva 27 Switzerland	Technical collaboration and grants for development of service programmes and information materials, provision of supplies and equipment, evaluation, and contraceptive research.
WHO Regional Office for Africa P.O. Box No. 6 Brazzaville Congo	
WHO Regional Office for the Americas/Pan American Sanitary Bureau 525 23rd Street, N.W. Washington, DC 20037 USA	
WHO Regional Office for the Eastern Mediterranean P.O. Box 1517 Alexandria 21511 Egypt	

Agency	Principal type(s) of assistance
WHO Regional Office for Europe 8 Scherfigsvej 2100 Copenhagen Denmark	
WHO Regional Office for South-East Asia World Health House Indraprastha Estate Mahatma Gandhi Road New Delhi—110002 India	
WHO Regional Office for the Western Pacific P.O. Box 2932 Manila 2801 Philippines	

In addition to the organizations listed in this annex, support may be available from a number of governmental and intergovernmental agencies. For a more complete listing of sources of assistance, see LEWISON, D. Sources of population and family planning assistance, *Population reports*, Series J, No. 26 (1983); and UNITED NATIONS POPULATION FUND, *Guide to sources of international population assistance*, 5th ed., New York, 1988.

Annex 2. Sample preoperative and postoperative instructions to clients (oral and written)

Written preoperative and postoperative instructions should be provided for literate and illiterate clients. They are especially important in helping women to recognize complications and in providing information on where to go if they occur. The staff should review the instructions with each client before surgery; the postoperative instructions should also be given just before the client leaves the facility.

Brief written instructions specific to each facility will need to be developed and pretested with clients. These should be written in the local language using terms that the clients can easily understand. The sample instructions below indicate what information should be given to clients.

What you should know about your sterilization operation

This leaflet contains important information that you need to know. It tells you how to prepare for your sterilization operation and to take care of yourself afterwards.

Remember, sterilization is a surgical procedure. It is meant to be permanent. After sterilization, you will no longer be able to get pregnant. If you have any questions or doubts, talk to the clinic staff. We are here to help you.

Before going to the clinic:

1. Do not eat or drink anything for eight hours before the operation. You will be able to eat and drink after the operation.

2. Before going to the clinic for the operation, have a bath. Carefully wash the navel, belly, and genital area using soap.

3. Wear clean loose clothing.

4. Arrange for a family member or friend to come to the clinic to help you home after the operation.

When you return home:

1. Rest for one or two days at home. You will probably be able to resume most of your normal activities within 3–5 days. Avoid heavy work or lifting for one week. This will help the wound heal.
2. Do not let the bandage get wet for 1–2 days.
3. Take the medicine provided by the clinic.
4. You may have sex as soon as it is comfortable for you. This is usually about one week after the operation.
5. Avoid pulling, scratching, or otherwise irritating the wound.
6. It is important for you to know what is normal following your surgery. There will probably be some pain and swelling around the wound; it may also be somewhat discoloured (bruised). This is normal and should not worry you.
7. Return to the clinic or notify the doctor or health worker if you have any of the following danger signals or if you notice any unusual body changes:
   - Fever within one week of the operation (over 38.0 °C or 100.4 °F).
   - A pain in your belly that does not go away or that becomes worse.
   - Bleeding or pus oozing from the wound.
   - Signs that you may be pregnant—a missed period, stomach pains, or dark or spotty bleeding between periods. Watch for these signs at any time after the operation. They may mean the operation has failed, and you may be pregnant. This could be dangerous for you.

   For any of these problems, you should telephone or go to the following location for medical care without delay:

   ____

   ____

   ____

   (add appropriate address)

Telephone number:

Annex 3. Minilaparotomy kit available from UNICEF

All of the items listed below can be ordered as one single kit (Tubal ligation kit, abdominal, UNICEF catalogue number 9950050) that can be obtained from UNICEF, UNICEF Plads, Freeport, DK 2100, Copenhagen, Denmark.

Item description	*Quantity*	*UNICEF catalogue number*
Forceps, tissue, Babcock, 20 cm	1	0736500
Instrument/dressing tray, covered, 310 × 195 × 63 mm	1	0276500
Surgeon's gloves, latex, size 6–6.5	12 pairs	0328000
Surgeon's gloves, latex, size 7, reusable	24 pairs	0328500
Surgeon's gloves, latex, size 7–7.5	24 pairs	0329000
Surgeon's gloves, latex, size 8, reusable	12 pairs	0329500
Towel clamp, Jones, 9 cm	4	0712100
Forceps, dressing, spring-type, 155 mm	1	0721000
Forceps, haemostat, straight, Rochester-Péan, 160 mm	4	0727500
Forceps, hysterectomy, straight, Péan, 220 mm	4	0728500
Forceps, haemostat, curved, mosquito, Halstead, 125 mm	2	0730000
Forceps, tissue, spring-type, 1 × 2 teeth, 145 mm	1	0737000
Forceps, tissue, fenestrated jaw, Duval, 145 mm	1	0739000

Item description	*Quantity*	*UNICEF catalogue number*
Forceps, uterine, tenaculum, Duplay, 280 mm	1	0740000
Needle holder, straight, narrow-jaw, Mayo, 180 mm	1	0743600
Knife handle, surgical, for minor surgery, size 3	1	0745000
Knife blade, surgical, for minor surgery, size 10 (5 per pack)	10 packs	0746000
Needle, suture, abdominal, Keith, straight	2 packs	0758600
Needle, suture, 3/8 circle, round point, size 12 (6 per pack)	2 packs	0759345
Retractor, general operating, Langenbeck, 60 × 20 mm	1	0768940
Retractors, abdominal, Richardson-Eastman (2 per set)	1 set	0767750
Scissors, surgical, straight, 145 mm	1	0774500
Scissors, tonsil, curved, Metzenbaum, baby, 150 mm	1	0774650
Speculum, vaginal, bi-valve, Graves, small	1	0777000
Speculum, vaginal, bi-valve, Graves, medium	1	0777500

Annex 4. Equipment for laparoscopic sterilization services

It is not possible to produce a standard list of equipment for laparoscopy procedures, as discussed earlier in Chapter 16. Nevertheless, the list below provides an example of the instruments and equipment that are needed to perform a typical laparoscopy procedure, using a single-puncture technique and clips or bands:

- Insufflation apparatus
- Carbon dioxide cylinder
- Laparoscope
- Fibre-optic light source with cable
- Veress needle
- Trocar and cannula
- Band or clip applicator
- Supply of bands or clips
- Uterine manipulator
- Cervical tenaculum
- Spare parts for light source

Additional instruments would be needed for procedures involving electrocoagulation. Other items that are generally recommended include spare parts for the insufflator for routine maintenance of the unit, and additional instruments for diagnostic procedures.

The addresses of the principal manufacturers of laparoscopic equipment may be obtained from the *Medical Device Register*, Volumes 1 and 2, 1989 (published by Medical Device Register Inc., 655 Washington Boulevard, Stamford, CT 06901, USA). Some of these manufacturers offer complete laparoscopy kits, while others offer only accessories and specific items, such as optical systems. For more information, contact the manufacturer directly.

Annex 5. Guidelines for developing and using client medical record and periodic summary report forms for female sterilization services

An example of a client medical record form is given below; this form is currently being used by government service providers in the Dominican Republic. The type of information that should be included on the client medical record form should be determined according to local conditions and needs. The following items are recommended for inclusion (WFHAAVSC, 1988):

1. **Client identification information**, including name, address, serial number, etc.
2. **Demographic information**, including age, marital status, etc.
3. **Client assessment/counselling information**, including reasons for requesting female sterilization.
4. **Informed-consent form**, properly completed (see page 69).
5. **Preoperative medical assessment**, including medical history, physical examination, vital signs, laboratory test results, etc.
6. **Medicines administered**, including doses and times given.
7. **Details of the surgical procedure**, including type of anaesthesia, surgical approach, method of occlusion, etc.
8. **Complications and outcomes of complications.**
9. **Postoperative and discharge notes.**
10. **Follow-up data.**

Some services find it useful to compile summary reports of certain details taken from the medical record forms of all clients who were served during a particular period. The type of information that is summarized will depend on local conditions, interests, and needs, but usually includes age and parity of clients, surgical approach used, method of tubal occlusion, type of anaesthesia, and complications. An example of a periodic summary report form, also used by service sites in the Dominican Republic, is given below.

It should be noted that coding boxes are provided for certain details given in the client medical record form, and that these coding boxes correspond to the columns in the periodic summary report. This allows for quick and easy transfer of information.

Sample medical record form for female sterilization services, as used in the Dominican Republic

1. Date of procedure ☐☐ ☐☐ ☐☐
   Day Month Year
2. Name of client ________________ 3. Client no .... ☐☐☐ A
4. Address:
5. Client's age in completed years .... ☐☐ B
6. Marital status: 1. Single 2. Married 3. Living in union 4. Widowed 5. Divorced/Separated
7. Education: 0. None 1. Primary 2. Intermediate 3. Secondary 4. University 5. Other (specify)
8. Number of living children .... ☐☐ C
9. Contraceptive method mainly used in past 3 months .... ☐ D
   (before conception for postabortion and postpartum cases)
   0. None 1. Pills 2. IUD 3. Subdermal implants 4. Injectables 5. Condoms 6. Spermicides 7. Other (specify)
10. Primary reason for requesting VSC procedure
    1. Desires no more children 2. Medical 3. Economic 4. Other (specify)

PREOPERATIVE CLINICAL INFORMATION

Medical History

	Yes	No		Yes	No		Yes	No
Heart disease	☐	☐	Psychiatric condition	☐	☐	Allergy to medication	☐	☐
Hypertension	☐	☐	Active tuberculosis	☐	☐	Pelvic inflammatory disease	☐	☐
Anaemia	☐	☐	Vaginal disorders	☐	☐	Pelvic/abdominal surgery	☐	☐
Diabetes	☐	☐	Bladder disorders	☐	☐			
Convulsive disorders	☐	☐	Bleeding disorders	☐	☐			

Drugs being taken ____________________________

Comments:

Obstetric History gravida ____ para ____ abortions ____

Date of last menses (month/day/year) __________

Date last pregnancy completed (month/day/year) __________

Physical Examination

Blood pressure ____ / ____ Pulse ____ Weight ____

Nutritional status:	1. Normal	2. Abnormal (describe)
Cardiorespiratory system:	1. Normal	2. Abnormal (describe)
Abdomen:	1. Normal	2. Abnormal (describe)

Pelvic Examination

External genitalia, vagina, cervix:	1. Normal	2. Abnormal (describe)
Uterine position:	1. Anteverted	2. Retroverted 3. Midline
Uterine size:	1. Normal	2. Enlarged or abnormal (describe)
Adnexa:	1. Normal	2. Abnormal (describe)
Uterine mobility:	1. Mobile	2. Fixed

Additional notes:

INTRAOPERATIVE INFORMATION

11. Timing of surgical contraception .... ☐ E

1. Immediate postpartum
2. Late postpartum
3. Postabortion
4. With caesarean section
5. Interval

12. Bladder emptied:
1. Voided before surgery
2. Catheterized
3. Bladder not emptied

Vital signs during surgery:

	Time	Pulse	Blood pressure	Respiratory rate
Preoperative				
During the operation				
Immediately postoperatively				

13. Anaesthesia .... ☐ F

1. Local only
2. Local with analgesia and/or sedation
3. Regional only (spinal, epidural, caudal)
4. Regional with analgesia and sedation
5. General—not intubated
6. General—intubated

	Drug	Dosage	Duration	Route
Anaesthesia				
Analgesia				

14. Surgical approach .... ☐ G

1. Laparotomy
2. Minilaparotomy
3. Laparoscopy
4. Other (specify)

15. Method of tubal occlusion .... ☐ H

1. Ring
2. Ligation with resection
3. Ligation without resection
4. Fimbriectomy
5. Salpingectomy
6. Clip
7. Other (specify)

16. Size of incision (cm) .... ☐ ☐ I

17. Duration of procedure

Time of incision _____ Time of closure _____

Total in minutes .... ☐ ☐ J

18. Procedure-associated complications and events .... ☐ K_1

0. None
1. Uterine perforation
2. Perforation or other injury to bladder
3. Perforation or other injury to intestine
4. Other organ injury
5. Major blood vessel injury
6. Life-threatening cardiorespiratory event
7. Other (specify)

☐ K_2

(Identify more than one if necessary; however, code only the two most important.)

Comments and details:

19. Surgical events .... ☐ L_1

0. Incomplete procedure
1. Difficulty finding tubes
2. Adhesions
3. Ovarian cysts
4. Inflamed tubes
5. Pregnancy
6. Difficulty penetrating peritoneal cavity
7. Other (specify)

☐ L_2

(Identify more than one if necessary; however, code only the two most important.)

Comments and details:

POSTOPERATIVE INFORMATION

Vital signs after surgery:

Time	Pulse	Blood pressure	Respiratory rate

20. Postoperative complications detected before discharge .... ☐ M_1

0. None
1. Pelvic infection
2. Wound infection and/ or haematoma
3. Urinary tract infection
4. Fever
5. Haemorrhage or abnormal bleeding
6. Life-threatening cardiorespiratory event
7. Severe abdominal pain
8. Other (specify)

☐ M_2

(Identify more than one if necessary; however, code only the two most important.)

If there are no complications, go to question 21.

Comments and details:

Treatment of complications:

Blood or plasma transfusion Yes No
Unintended surgery Yes No

Comments and details (describe other relevant treatment; for example, antibiotics):

21. Date of discharge ____________________

Number of nights client spent at facility postoperative .... ☐ N

22. Discharge status .... ☐ O

1. Discharged well
2. Discharged with home treatment
3. Referred to another facility for management of complications
4. Deceased

If patient transferred, give name of institution and state reason for transfer.

Other postoperative notes (include name of person recording information):

FOLLOW-UP INFORMATION

23. Source of follow-up information .... ☐ P

1. Clinic visit (spontaneous)
2. Clinic visit (after home visit)
3. Home visit
4. Other clinic/hospital report
5. Other (specify)

Date of follow-up ______________________________

24. Complications after discharge .... ☐ Q_1

0. None
1. Pelvic infection
2. Wound infection and/or haematoma
3. Urinary tract infection
4. Fever not associated with above complications (38 °C or more for 3 or more days)
5. Haemorrhage or abnormal bleeding ☐ Q_2
6. Life-threatening cardio-respiratory event
7. Severe abdominal pain not associated with above complications
8. Other (specify)

(Identify more than one if necessary; however, code only the two most important.)

If no complications are recorded, go to question 25.

Comments and details:

Treatment of complications:

Blood or plasma transfusion	Yes	No
Surgery	Yes	No
Hospitalization	Yes	No

Comments and details (describe other relevant treatment; for example, antibiotics):

Date this information recorded ______________________________

25. Current condition of client .... ☐ R

1. Complete recovery
2. Still receiving treatment
3. Referred to another facility for management of complications
4. Deceased

If patient referred to another health care facility, give name of institution and state reason for referral.

Other notes:

Sample summary report form for female sterilization services, as used in

Name of institution: ______________________________

Reporting period ☐☐ Month ☐☐ Year ☐ Region ☐☐ Province

A	B	C	D	E	F	G	H	I	J	K	L
Client number	Age	Contraceptive method	No. of surviving children	Timing of procedure	Anaesthesia	Surgical approach	Method of occlusion	Incision length (cm)	Duration of procedure (min)	Procedure-associated complications	Surgical events

the Dominican Republic

☐☐

Municipality

M	N	O	P	Q	R	
Postoperative complications	No. of nights hospitalized	Discharge status	Source of follow-up	Complications after discharge	Current condition	COMMENTS

Harris Methodist
Health Sciences Library
1301 Pennsylvania Ave.
Fort Worth, TX 76104